DANCES WITH WEREWOLVES

I'm naked, cold and completely helpless.

My hands and neck are shackled to the wall of the cell with heavy iron manacles. The bonds hold me in an uncomfortable position between standing and squatting and my aching thighs tremble with the effort.

Above me, a pipe drips water onto my head. It soaks my hair and trickles down my face, into my eyes and over my body, pooling in soft splashes at my feet. Shivering, I gasp at the shocking cold. It feels like drowning on my feet.

I shake my head wildly, spraying droplets everywhere. But I can't escape the relentless dripping water and I'm drenched again in seconds. I know they're watching me, waiting for me to break.

After a few hours of this I will surrender. I will sign what they want me to sign.

I will confess.

DANCES WITH WEREWOLVES

Niki Flynn

First published in 2007 by
Virgin Books
Thames Wharf Studios
Rainville Rd
London W6 9HA

A catalogue record of this book is available from the British
Library

ISBN 978 0 7535 1228 9

The paper used in this book is a natural, recyclable product
made from wood grown in sustainable forests. The
manufacturing process conforms to the regulations of the
country of origin.

Typeset by TW Typesetting, Plymouth, Devon
Printed and bound by CPI Bookmarque, Croydon CR0 4TD

1 3 5 7 9 10 8 6 4 2

For my parents,
who always encouraged me to follow my dreams,
even if they'd be shocked by where those dreams
have led me.

CONTENTS

ACKNOWLEDGEMENTS

My first thanks must go to Jeoffry, who read an early draft with the ruthlessness of a fellow writer. Thanks also to Chris and Pablo and Mija, kinky friends who tried to see it through vanilla eyes for me. And of course Cameron, who had to read it in its worst stages.

Special thanks to the members of my Yahoo group, who first suggested this memoir. Unfortunately, the nice folks at Yahoo deleted the group the day I received the proofs for this book.

To Ramsey Campbell, for being unnerved. Yes, that *is* a compliment from the man who gave me so many sleepless nights.

To David Westfield, for letting me play rock star for a day, even if I did have the worst hangover ever the next morning.

To my sister, the kinkiest boy I know.

To all the friends, tormentors, models, filmmakers and photographers who have helped me live out my fantasies.

Most importantly, thanks to all the fans and viewers. This book wouldn't exist without them.

NOTE:
Some names and identifying details have been changed to protect the privacy of the people involved.

Visit the author's website
www.nikiflynn.com

PLAYING ON THE EDGE

There will be censorship.

I say this from experience, both as a writer and as a reviewer. Show me a new medium and I'll guarantee it will attract censorship as soon as it becomes popular (or, in some instances, once it attracts public notice). In my lifetime alone this has befallen comic books, videos and the Internet, not to mention old favourites such as films and books. Indeed, not so long ago this very book would have been unpublishable in English outside Paris. In the 50s, horror comics aimed at adults apparently had to be stopped, and so they were in Britain by the Children and Young Persons (Harmful Publications) Bill, encouraged by a newspaper outcry under headlines such as 'Now Ban This Filth That Poisons Our Children' and 'Make Bonfires of Them' (the comics, not the children), along with a persistent media claim that a gunman called Alan Poole had been influenced by his collection of hundreds of horror comics, although in fact he owned just a solitary comic, a Western one eventually described in Parliament as 'not very alarming'.

A media campaign that uses an unexamined scare story or a single unrepresentative crime to whip up hysteria until the government feels forced to bring in extra censorship – it's a recurring set of events. In the early 80s it was the turn of the nasty: while the term was coined by a publicist to sell horror fiction, it was hijacked to describe videos the public was supposed to find objectionable. The *Daily Mail* urged 'Ban the Sadist

Videos' and clearly had the ear of Bernard Braine, who referred in the House of Lords to 'a grave and growing social evil which no civilised or caring society would tolerate ... a filthy and pernicious trade' (which is to say, making and distributing horror films he didn't like).

All this (along with earlier media tirades that blamed the Industrial Revolution, the music hall, the bicycle and – 'a grave danger to the community, responsible for the downfall of many young people' – silent cinema for the collapse of society) may be history, but some of us lived elements of it. In 1969 my parents' house was raided when I advertised a copy of de Sade's *120 Days of Sodom* for sale, while in the 90s Her Majesty's Customs confiscated one of the *Men Behind the Sun* videos (a series of fictional reconstructions of Japanese atrocities in Manchuria) and sent me a small nastily duplicated scrap of paper warning of the legal dangers of importing 'obscene' material. I suspect that the sender may have been the kind of petty bureaucrat into whose unyielding grip identity cards and a blind faith in computer information will deliver us. The film would certainly be released uncut here now, as most of the nasties have been (three of them rated as suitable for anybody over fourteen to watch), and you can buy the exact same unexpurgated translation of de Sade in any major British bookshop. The other recurring truth about censorship (sometimes exerted by the marketplace, the reason why David McGillivray's excellent anti-censorship magazine *Scapegoat* lasted for just a single issue) is that it tends to go away. Since the turn of this century the British board has taken the view that films rated suitable for adults should be cut only for exceptional reasons, which will be specified on the BBFC's website. One kind of film that has continued to bother the board is a central issue of the present book.

It did even after the R18 certificate allowed hardcore sex films to be legally released. In 2000 the board refused to pass *A Caning for Miss Granger* (a video in which the eponymous office worker is also spanked and strapped, if relatively mildly), citing as unacceptable 'the portrayal of any sexual activity, whether real or simulated, which involves lack of consent'. The press release went on to say that 'The Board's Guidelines prohibit the infliction of pain or physical harm, real or (in a sexual context) simulated ... The Board concluded that the work both promotes the idea that pleasure may be taken from inflicting pain upon another person and clearly shows, with some relish, actual pain and physical harm. In doing so it goes some way beyond what might be regarded as "mild consensual activity". The Board does not feel that the problems can be usefully addressed by cutting since the difficulty with this work lies not only in the great number of specific visual images, but with the overall theme of sexual pleasure being derived from imposing pain on a coerced victim. The work is therefore not suitable for classification.'

On the whole the Board is lenient towards spankings embedded in mainstream movies, including the episode in *The Fearless Vampire Killers* where the director watches through a keyhole as his then wife is spanked by Alfie Bass, surely one of the most extraordinary confessional moments in all cinema. As far as hardcore goes, though, has anything changed? Let me save the answer for the end. Meanwhile, it would be naïve of me to suggest that a time will ever come when such material won't be attacked or, if you prefer, misunderstood. Some years ago I wrote a survey of several dozen British videos in the genre, and felt bound to allow for reservations. Aren't the films catering to male fantasies? (Of course they are, but not exclusively by any means.) Don't they, and indeed porn in general, degrade women? (Quite apart from all the male gay porn this recurring objection excludes from the argument, would it be perverse to suggest that the idea itself degrades the models by reducing them to mere representatives of their gender, denying them individuality and choice?) Can the participants really be consenting to their treatment? As you'll see as you read on, even Niki Flynn used to wonder (although it's typical of her that she set out to discover the truth by experience). She reassures us – certainly me – in her admirably honest reminiscences, which offer more insight into this kind of play than I've ever read elsewhere.

Ms Flynn begins with reminiscences of the solitary spanko's (or, as the spellchecker insists I should have written, the solitary spinach's) guilty youth – the sense of exclusion, the contradictory desires to pass for ordinary and to yield to the secret self. I ought to say that, like the Nexus novelist Fiona Locke, she has a good deal of wry fun with this, not least because it's so sharply observed – especially the many paradoxes inherent in it – and the same is the case with some of her accounts of filming. You'll learn of the ideal dress for such occasions (and how it isn't always respected). You'll read where Rosaleen Young (an auteur in this field if there ever was one) has been known to direct her films from (if I may be permitted a parenthesis so as not to finish with a preposition). You'll observe Niki's search for the best description of her activities: stuntgirl seems to ring true, but I'd suggest performance artist as well. You may be comforted by some of the anecdotes from behind the scenes (confirmed by extras on the DVDs), and you'll learn how fearsome the Strap of Joy proved to be, and how hard it is to dismember a bear. However, this is by no means just a book of informative fun. Her psychological scrutiny illuminates places some readers (even though any buyer of this book will presumably have kinks in common with the author) may find very dark.

Let's confront the central truth. Niki Flynn doesn't play for the audience, however much of one there is: she does it to explore her own fantasies. I believe she will take it as a compliment that I find some of her films genuinely unnerving, and on occasion very hard to watch. Her accounts herein of her more extreme experiences are simultaneously harrowing and reassuring, and there's a remarkable moment among the extras on the DVD of *Stalin 2* that more than bears them out. She's interviewed before and after a particularly severe scene, and in the latter section of the interview she has plainly attained an extraordinary psychological state. Since she uses the word herself in the course of the book, I'll presume to suggest that she achieved a form of transcendence.

I referred in passing to her audience. Some readers may feel this needs to be taken more into account if not regarded with suspicion. I don't believe the response of an audience can be easily controlled or predicted. I've found this not just with my own fiction but in other instances, perhaps most strikingly when a fellow judge of a literary prize objected to a scene in one of the competing novels (an episode in which a nun who has just left the convent is embarrassed by her underwear while shopping in a boutique) as a male fantasy, demeaning to women, until I revealed that I'd identified the anonymous co-authors, one of whom was an ex-nun drawing on her own experience. We may also assume that Marilyn French intended the spanking reminiscence in *The Women's Room* to outrage her feminist audiences, but a significant number of readers take it quite another way. As for censoring material on the chance that it may provoke non-consensual imitation, I offer the alternative possibility that consuming it may be the only outlet the viewer needs, and that suppression may leave viewers no outlet for their fantasies except real life. But shouldn't material that's perceived as potentially dangerous be outlawed just in case it causes crime? What if the material prevents crime by allowing the viewer to be content with fantasy?

While Niki Flynn's English and American films are as much fun for the participants as for the audience (I was amused and delighted to find books of mine figuring as props in two of them), her European work is closer to the edge yet edges closer to relatively mainstream genres. The *Stalin* films are so intense in their recreation of the nightmare of totalitarianism that they're seldom even erotic, though disturbing when they veer that way. In their sense of panic they're closer to the horror film, where terror is often inextricable from an erotic element. (The Lupus film *The Orphan* – not one of Niki's – recalls Hans Andersen in its icy cruelty, but no angels are flown in to save the day.) It isn't surprising that Niki Flynn admires the films of David Lynch, in some of which – *Blue Velvet*, *Lost Highway* – eroticism and terror are inseparable and inescapable. As a horror writer I often have to assure interviewers that, rather than striving to be scary, my fiction tries to convey how the themes and observations make me feel, and it's clear from her starker work that Niki Flynn believes in undergoing the situations she depicts, not just in acting them. She brings to them, or discovers in them, a sense of real dread. Her *Stalin* films are also related to the Women In Prison genre, a form originated by John Cromwell's 1950 movie *Caged* and sometimes redeemed from disreputability (if one feels it needs redemption) by a political subtext, for instance in the Japanese *Female Convict Scorpion* series. On the other hand, politics are precisely the problem (if there is one) with her film *The Spy*, condemned by some as an unacceptable fantasy. You might expect kinky folk to be more tolerant of other people's kinks, but it doesn't always work like that: try calling a spanko a masochist, or confusing CP with BDSM, and you're likely to provoke the kind of reaction you'd meet if you mistook a science fiction fan for a fantasy reader. In *The Spy* the contentious element is the setting of an interrogation fantasy in a fascist regime some find uncomfortably similar to Nazism (even though the insignia on the armbands resemble symbols in a futuristic film about dictatorship far more than swastikas). Why is this objectionable? In *The Night Porter*, after all, Nazism is explicitly the basis of an erotic, not to say perverse, relationship. It may be argued that *The Night Porter*, unlike the films that were stimulated by it, is about eroticism rather than erotic in itself, but the present book proves this not to be the case. The truth is surely that it's impossible to predict the effect of any text, written or visual, on every member of its audience. Look at the Bible. Look at the Koran.

I ended my rant about censorship with the refusal of an R18, but we've moved on. Last year *An American Brat in London*, starring none other than Niki Flynn, gained the certificate, if in a version somewhat re-edited before submission by the director. As I write, her latest British film *Trial by Ordeal* appears to have been passed uncut with the certificate, confirming the precedent that greater severity can be allowed at R18 (and indeed can be the only reason for the rating). This seems to establish that such material will be safe from any proposed new censorship, however intensively that may be campaigned for. I hope none of her work will be threatened. Even if she's had to don a *nom de fessée*, Niki Flynn has certainly earned her fame. Here's to more.

Ramsey Campbell
Wallasey, Merseyside
17 May 2007

My fear is my substance
and probably the best part of me.

Franz Kafka

1. PROFESSIONAL VICTIM

'Give me pain, Niki!'

I screw my face into an expression of agony as the camera clicks and I pretend that the hand pressing into my bottom is smacking me. I'm already sore and tender from the real spanking Heather gave me a few minutes ago. The stills are done afterwards, recreating the video we've just shot. And yes, they're usually faked.

Viewers sometimes complain that a girl's bottom is already red in the stills that allegedly show the beginning of the punishment. There's really no way around it. You can't shoot the stills and the video at the same time. Otherwise you hear the camera and see the flash during the scene.

They also assume that this is a regular day job, that we turn up at the studio every day to shoot one clip and then go home. In reality I shoot about a dozen clips in a day, so it's not surprising that my bottom is bruised by the end. Viewers don't realise that a ten-minute clip can take three times that long to film. Or that it takes an hour or two just to set up the lighting and props. Or that the 'new' update on the website was probably shot several months ago. Companies produce huge amounts of content in one go and then dole it out piecemeal.

'Raise your hand, Heather,' Mike directs, snapping away. 'That's good, now lift her skirt.'

I feign shock and outrage as she lifts my pleated school skirt and positions her hand across my white cotton knickers. This is the usual sequence. Over the skirt, over the knickers, then on the bare. In a video it provides a warm-up, gradually getting my bottom used to being smacked. Many people like the slow progression and it can help disguise the fact that I'm already marked. I don't like it myself; it's inauthentic. And I'm all about authenticity.

Posed stills are nowhere near as much fun as movies. I want the real thing; I want the ritual, the scolding, the anticipation. It's an elaborate dance with precise choreography. Anxiety, exposure, vulnerability, surrender, pain, endurance, bliss . . . Like ballet, it looks effortless. But, like ballet, the cornerstone is pain.

I love being paired with a skilled top who knows how to intimidate me and has an answer for all my backchat. No matter how much I resist, the object of the game is to lose. That's what the viewers are paying to see and it's what I want too. I crave the moment of surrender, the moment when I finally give in and have to submit to the sting of a firm hand or a cane across my bare bottom. It's what I live for.

I don't really like the term 'spanking model'. But 'actress' is too pretentious. And while I get a kick out of calling myself a porn star, I don't actually have sex on camera. I don't have sex for money at all, though I respect those who do. However, what I do is undeniably 'intended to arouse', so I suppose technically I'm a sex worker.

Whatever you call me, I get paid to be spanked, paddled, caned and whipped on camera. And I love what I do. Is there anything better than getting paid for doing what you love? Kind of like a nymphomaniac getting paid for sex. It hardly seems fair to call it a job. I don't do it for the money, but there's an added thrill in being paid for it. So you can call me a whore too. Really. I like it.

'More reaction, Niki!'

I arch on Heather's lap, my eyes wide as I crane round, reacting with exaggerated horror as she raises her hand high above my backside. When she pulls my knickers down I reach back as if to stop her. She pins my wrist against my back and I grit my teeth when I feel her hand on my bottom. We vary our positions and the camera records our efforts. It's more work than you'd imagine.

The headmistress's office is actually a corner of Mike's garage. A bad *trompe-l'oeil* bookshelf covers the wall behind us, and I'm surrounded by light-stands, soft boxes and slave flashes that blind me every time they go off. The place is a deathtrap of electrical cords and tripods and the room still stinks of burned plastic where one of the makeshift reflectors melted against a light bulb.

Welcome to my world.

'Right, that's enough OTK.'

Over the knee is everyone's favourite spanking position. It's just so intimate and humbling, especially for a grown woman dressed as a schoolgirl. The vulnerability turns me on like nothing else.

Mike lowers the camera. 'What did you use next, Heather?'

'The leather paddle and then the cane.'

'No, it was just the cane,' I remind her. 'The leather paddle was in the French maid scene.'

Heather laughs. 'Oh, right.'

Sometimes it's hard to remember what you've just done. Especially when you're on the eighth vignette of the day. It took ten minutes just to get the white balance right for the stills and that's quite long enough to lose track. Clips like this are all improvisation, so there's no script to refer to. Not that you can cram much plot into a five-minute clip anyway; they're 90 per cent action.

We reposition ourselves. The headmistress looms over me, flexing the cane menacingly while I chew my lip and look worried. It's hard to resist the urge to ham it up with campy, melodramatic expressions. It's like filming a silent movie.

Another shot and our eyes lock. Heather looks so earnest it's hard to keep a straight face. Mike waits too long to push the button and we break into giggles and spoil the shot. He grumbles.

Trying again, I unfocus my eyes and look just above her eyebrows to avoid making her laugh again. Heather and I can never make eye contact without cracking up.

Click. Click. Click.

I stretch out over the desk and we re-enact the caning. I cringe in anticipation. I arch my back as she presses the cane against my cheeks. I kick. A fan told me once that I have the best kick in the business. I open my mouth wide as though howling in pain. I grit my teeth. This is where it gets tedious. There are only so many faces you can pull.

'Hang on,' Heather says. 'Weren't your knickers on the desk for this part?'

I have no idea.

We look over at Mike, who shrugs. 'No one'll notice,' he says dismissively.

He'd be surprised. You wouldn't believe some of the things guys pick up on. There are some serious pedants and fantasists out there who spot every continuity glitch. They're impossible to satisfy, but they're some of my favourite correspondents. I find their discernment extremely erotic.

'OK, Niki, you ready for some impact shots?'

I groan. I hate impact shots. Most models do. They're so unflattering.

Heather positions the cane and Mike counts to three.

'One, two, three—'

WHACK!

These are actual strokes. And when the timing is right the shots are dramatic. They make you realise just how powerful an implement the cane really is. Even a hand causes the cheeks to flatten out like a rubber ball squashed against a window, but the cane creates a wave that ripples away from the line of impact. We also call them 'pancake shots'. It's the least attractive image you'll ever see of a girl's bottom. But the guys seem to like them. There's certainly no way to fake those shots. After four or five of these, I'm starting to hurt again.

I have a high pain threshold and I can take a lot of punishment – especially with the cane, my favourite implement. But it's not the caning itself I get off on; it's the aftermath. I don't actually like *being* caned; I like having *been* caned.

The other side of the pain is where I want to be; that's where I find euphoria. Pain is the process I have to endure to get there. And when all the elements are right, I can fly.

WHACK!

'Oww!'

'You all right, Niki?' Heather asks.

'Yeah, I'm fine.'

'Use your safeword if you need to.'

The safeword is my code for 'stop!' It's the signal to halt a scene that's getting too intense. 'No', 'please' and 'stop' won't work; protest is a key element of the punishment fantasy. In my world 'no' often *does* mean 'yes', so the safeword has to be something I'd never ordinarily say, like 'red' or 'kingfisher' or even simply 'safeword'.

One girl I know uses 'ouch'. If she's OK she says 'oww,' but 'ouch' means it's getting too much. The bottom is always in control, you see. I like 'cut!' myself, though I can usually survive until there's a natural break in the action.

But for now it's back to reality. I have to pace myself for the rest of the shoot. I'm eager to finish the stills so we can get to the next video. I have a bratty comeback I'm dying to spring on Heather.

I'm notorious for putting my darkest fantasies on film and I'm known for unglamorous roles and edgy movies. I embrace intense scenarios many people won't go near. Military interrogations and prison abuse. And yet the school kink is a vital part of my sexuality, of who I am.

For me there's nothing like an authentic English school caning. Six of the best. Skirt up, knickers down. I've been caned by more headmasters and headmistresses than I can count. I can knot a school tie blindfolded. And I've had 'sir' and 'miss' drilled into me so thoroughly that it slips out occasionally in vanilla company. It's a tiny taste of the school life I never had in America.

'Well done,' Mike says, satisfied at last. 'Now, for the next scene . . . Heather, let's have you in your nurse's uniform. Niki, did you say you had a straitjacket?'

WARNING!

This is an adult site dealing with consensual corporal punishment of adults. **Access by minors is strictly forbidden.** If you are a minor or if this subject offends you then please click here to exit.

All models are over the age of 18. We are in no way suggesting otherwise. Neither this site nor its owners condones the corporal punishment of minors, nor the depiction of minors in any media for sexual gratification.

All images displayed on this site comply with **18 USC §2257**.

We strongly support parental controls on the Internet. If you want to block this site, please contact one of the following filtering systems:

CyberPatrol SurfWatch NetNanny SafeSurf CyberSitter

2. STRANGE LITTLE GIRL

All my life I've been drawn to the dark side. I was a weird kid. (Weren't we all?) Painfully shy and introverted, I hid inside my own little shell, trying not to be noticed. I was obsessed with horror movies. The nightmares they inspired only fuelled my dark imagination more. When the other girls played house, I wanted to be the ghost. Every house had one, I insisted. Their expressions said it all: *You are not like us. You are not normal.* So I learned to keep my bizarre ideas to myself.

In school I was a typical Ophelia wannabe, dressed all in black and romanticising death. Morbid fantasies consumed me. Lost in my own world, I imagined elaborate scenarios where I was kidnapped, punished, tied up, tortured, brainwashed, raped. Sometimes even killed.

Happy endings bored me. I needed to suffer in order to feel.

Throughout high school I had a recurring fantasy involving all the boys who had ever humiliated me. I wasn't 'cool' enough to enter their sphere. I was just a freaky girl in black who, while no different from a hundred thousand other freaky girls in black, was worthy only of their scorn. So I took the shame and made it my own.

In my fantasy I was wandering alone in the woods when they ambushed me. I ran, but they gave chase and caught me. They stripped me, tied my hands behind my back and whipped me.

After that they took turns violating me in every way I could imagine. When they'd had their fun, they killed me and dumped my body in the river.

It was an oddly sterile scene. There was never any dialogue. And I experienced the murder from a safe distance, as a ghost. I was a martyr and they were the wicked villains who had used and abused me. My conscience was clear.

Fear was my drug of choice. I thrived on scary movies, ghost stories and rollercoasters. I dreamed of playing the last girl left alive in a slasher film – the one who screams herself hoarse as she discovers her friends' bodies one by one. Naturally, she's the first one killed in the sequel.

There was just something about fear, helplessness and even violence that pushed certain buttons for me. Even as a child. I had no way of knowing they were budding sexual feelings; I just knew they made me feel strange in a way that wasn't entirely bad.

Like when I played the lead in an eighth-grade school play about a girl shipwrecked on an alien planet. In one scene the aliens captured me and tied me to a tree. 'Tighter,' I remember whispering to my co-stars. 'Make it look real.' No, it had nothing to do with Method acting, but that was my dirty little secret.

Fetishes are deeply personal. They're not something you choose. Nor can you 'cure' yourself of them. The road to sexual awareness is a rocky one, especially if what turns you on is different from what's considered 'normal'. Rejection and ridicule are powerful deterrents. It's no wonder some people live their whole lives in the closet, never sharing their fantasies with anyone.

Spanking in particular has always gotten a bad rap. Think of all the kinky spanking scenes you've seen in movies. How many portray it as a healthy, intimate act between sane and consenting adults? Sometimes it's characterised as a neurotic fixation on reliving childhood abuse, but more often it's comic relief. People laugh at the middle-aged civil servant in short trousers, getting his bottom smacked by a woman he's paid for the privilege. They love to mock such people when they get lampooned by the *News of the World*. Why? If they've never had an intimate confession to make to a partner, then I truly envy them.

As a child I was confused and conflicted by my reactions to certain scenes in movies and books. I remember an animated fairy tale that I saw once in school. My friends appreciated the damsel-in-distress scenario – but only the part where the princess was rescued by the handsome prince. That was where I lost interest. I didn't want her to be rescued. I felt cheated out of details of the kidnapping, the imprisonment and the unseen torments inflicted on her by the villain. He was much more appealing than the boring one-dimensional prince. My imagination ran wild, but I knew by then to keep my mouth shut.

Though I was a weird kid, I was a well-behaved one. Cruel classmates teased me and called me 'Goody Two Shoes'. The paddle was still in use when I was in school, but I never did anything bad enough to earn it. I was tempted, though. The gym teachers were zealous practitioners of corporal punishment and it would have been easy enough to get on the wrong side of them. I'd occasionally hear the loud CRACK! echoing through the halls as some unfortunate kid felt the board. I don't need to tell you the effect it had on me.

Eventually I found the signposts that led the way to others like me. The first was the movie *Videodrome*. I saw it around the time I entered puberty, when I was at my most conflicted. In one scene Nicki Brand is looking for some porn to get her in the mood. She finds a tape labelled 'Videodrome' and asks what it is. Max Renn nonchalantly replies, 'Torture. Murder.' She smiles. 'Sounds great.' 'Ain't exactly sex,' he warns her. But there's a gleam in Nicki's eye. 'Says who?'

Says who indeed. Nicki Brand was the first masochistic character I had ever encountered. And while she was only a character in a movie, she validated my preoccupation with being victimised. I related to her even more when she said she was 'made for that show' and went off to discover where it was filmed. Her self-assurance gave me courage. I wanted to be like that – confident in my unconventional desires. Embracing the lure of pain and not caring whether or not anyone else understood. I needed to know that such people could exist.

The next signpost was a roleplay experience like no other. Every Halloween the local fire department hosted a haunted house for the kids. When they asked for volunteers from my high school I knew I had found my dream job. I was sixteen. The high point was when the boy I was madly in love with played Freddy Krueger from *Nightmare on Elm Street*. I got to be his victim.

I wore a torn nightgown splattered with fake blood. Freddy attacked me and I screamed, dying again and again, night after night. I told him to be rough with me and gave him my standard line: 'Make it look real.' He did, oblivious to how much it was turning me on. I never wanted it to end. I'd go home every night with bruises and scratches from our struggles. Then I'd lie in bed, too keyed up to sleep but too self-conscious to relieve my frustration. I just couldn't bring myself to masturbate to fantasies about Freddy Krueger!

(Now, Hannibal Lecter on the other hand . . .)

As I distilled and refined my fetish, I realised that it wasn't death or even violence that turned me on. Ultimately it was power. There is nothing more erotic to me than power. And that most special privilege of the empowered: *discipline*.

Spankos speculate endlessly on what made us the way we are. Some blame it on corporal punishment at home and school. But there are just as many who can't trace it to any defining moment. I was spanked while growing up, but my adult fantasies couldn't be further from my childhood reality. Frankly, I think my obsession with fear and horror informed my sexuality more than any actual spanking did.

I read *Story of O* and other BDSM novels, but the traditional Master/slave relationship didn't resonate with me. I wasn't submissive. I wasn't aroused by pleasure. But I wasn't a true masochist like Nicki Brand either; I didn't actually like pain. So why was I so obsessed by the power dynamic, with pain such a crucial element? I felt just as lost as when I'd started my quest.

At last I found my Rosetta Stone. *Frank and I*. It's a classic Victorian novel about a girl – 'Frances' – who disguises herself as a boy – 'Frank'. She's adopted by a wealthy gentleman who wants to help the lad and see that he gets a proper education. He's also a strict disciplinarian and he discovers the secret when he orders Frank to drop his trousers for a birching. A confessed 'lover of the rod', he keeps the knowledge to himself, continuing to treat his young ward as a boy and administering punishment at every opportunity.

In one scene Frank's guardian decides not to birch the girl, as he thinks it will be more exciting to put her over his knee and spank her. Yes, yes, yes! Submitting to someone with the authority to punish me – *that* was what I wanted! I didn't have to be submissive; I just had to submit. And I didn't have to enjoy it; I just had to take it.

I was ecstatic at the discovery. Punishment had always fascinated me, but I had never realised anyone else found it sexually arousing. Now I knew where to channel my energies. And I thought I knew how to ask for what I wanted. I underlined every hot disciplinary passage and gave the book to my college boyfriend Roger. I assumed that it would hit the same bullseye for him.

'You find this sexy?' he asked, as though I'd given him a book on waste-disposal management.

'Well, not exactly sexy, but . . .' I should have known better.

Roger was a Christian who tolerated my atheism with pursed lips and the creepy warning that one day all the Christians would be taken off the earth, leaving me to face the lake of fire alone. One day he found my copy of the *Necronomicon*, having 'sensed its evil presence' while snooping around in my bedroom. After a discussion with his father, a self-styled demon hunter (I kid you not), Roger destroyed the book. Well, Lovecraft might have been flattered, but I was pretty pissed off. The relationship didn't last long.

In another clumsy attempt to reach out I wrote a cringeworthy essay called 'Mary Shelley, Sadomasochist'. Playing amateur psychoanalyst, I theorised that Shelley enjoyed making her virtuous female characters suffer in *Frankenstein*, symbolically destroying the image of the passive and subservient female she refused to be herself. I leaped at the chance to compare her Justine character to de Sade's tortured protagonist of the same name, suggesting that Shelley must have been a fan. (I wrote a lot of papers like that.) My pretentious effort earned me the devastating comment 'Imaginative but not exactly relevant'. Another failure.

I had no outlet for my fantasies and no one I could share them with. So I wrote stories, scribbling down my secret thoughts and squirreling them away under my mattress. I read them again and again, lying on my stomach with my panties pulled down to my knees as I got myself off. I had no interest in sex. My fantasies were only about spanking. I couldn't get aroused without thinking about it.

It was important for me that my disciplinarian got no sexual charge out of the act. I would cast my favourite actor as the businesslike authority figure who wouldn't be swayed by any tearful pleas. He wasn't sadistic; he was simply doing his job, for my own good. The emotional detachment was essential. As was my own genuine fear and dislike of the punishment. It was really just a variation on the rape fantasy. No guilt. No responsibility. Someone else was in control and there was no danger of rejection.

What I was doing with my hands had nothing to do with the scene I was playing out in my head. The sensations were wonderful, but they weren't happening to the girl in the fantasy. Kind of like having a massage while watching a movie. And picturing myself over a strict man's knee, having my bare bottom smacked, it wouldn't take me long to reach a shattering climax. Profound embarrassment followed the afterglow, but it never made me stop.

Some months later I panicked when I thought the pages under my mattress had been disturbed. Had my parents been snooping? Had they read my dirty stories? In a panic I burned them all and tried to convince myself that I wasn't a pervert. I could forget this sick fetish. I could be like other people.

I could be normal.

Hi Niki,

Just wanted to let you know that I really enjoyed seeing you caned in *Exchange Student*. How long did the marks last?

For your next movie, would you consider a scenario where you are suspended by your wrists nude for a whipping across your back? After this you would be caned again. I would suggest a whipping of 50 lashes and a caning of about 80–100 strokes. Think you can handle this?

Best regards,

Mr Ravenwood, USA

3. THE FIRST TIME

I was born kinky. My earliest memory is a dream I had when I was about five years old. It was very simple, very Freudian. I had wandered into the kingdom behind the sofa in my parents' den, where the king caught me. He stood over me in his red velvet robe and golden crown, scowling and shaking his finger. Then he sat down heavily on his throne, turned me over his knee and spanked me. My father was sitting in his big black recliner, reading. He watched impassively for a few seconds before turning back to his paper.

I woke up feeling as though I'd done something bad. I was deeply ashamed. I didn't understand why spanking fascinated me and I didn't understand why it felt wrong to be fascinated. I was embarrassed by the dream and terrified that my father had somehow seen it through my eyes. (This was a recurring delusion whenever I did things I knew he wouldn't approve of.) Guilt, shame and confusion plagued me for years.

The Net changed everything. I had just graduated from college when I typed 'spanking' into a search engine and discovered a whole new world. 'I am ONLINE!' I scrawled in my diary. 'And I also know now that I am truly, truly unhappy.'

My vanilla life was over, you see. And with it my vanilla relationship.

Once I found other spankos and realised that other people had fantasies complementary to mine, I knew I would never be able to bottle up my desires again. I was sick of lying to my partner and to myself. Sick of sacrificing my pleasure for his. I was wasting my time pretending to be someone I wasn't when there were others out there who wanted exactly what I wanted.

So I said goodbye forever to vanilla boyfriends and dived into the spanking scene.

I met kinky friends and went to kinky parties. I played with lots of people, but I didn't seriously consider doing it professionally until much later. Looking back now, it seems such an obvious path. The idea was hot; I just lacked the confidence. Besides, I didn't know anything about the pro side of things. I imagined the stereotypical sleazy porn mogul (I'll make you a star, baby!) who would take advantage of his naïve little ingénue, pushing her further than she wanted to go.

Not that I had any experience of mainstream porn films, mind you. I'd seen the cheesy softcore ones they showed late at night on cable TV. Occasionally there'd be a scene with some campy bondage or whipping but, even when they weren't caricatures, they were simply too lame to be arousing.

I saw my first real porn film with a group of friends in college. Long before I knew other spankos existed. You'll laugh at this, but, when the first penetration shot appeared on the screen, I was shocked.

'Oh my God,' I gasped. 'They're actually having sex!'

Everyone stared at me.

'Yeah . . . It's a porno.'

That was an instant education. I'd been expecting slightly more graphic simulation of what I'd seen in the softcore movies. It had never occurred to me that a porno was *actual sex*. My mind reeled as I made secret connections: if there were movies of real sex, might there also be movies of real spanking?

My sister Jessie was a year younger, but a lot more worldly wise. I'd stayed at home and gone to a local college on a drama scholarship, terrified of the prospect of being on my own around so many new people and having to share a room with a stranger. Jessie, my polar opposite, had gone to a university in another city, eager to party away from home. Her new friends introduced her to all kinds of interesting things. While I was getting secret thrills out of performing a scene from *Taming of the Shrew* and wishing my Petruchio would spank me, Jessie was discovering drugs and kinky sex. She also discovered my first fellow spanko.

On one of Jessie's weekends home, before the Net, I asked her to go with me to a porn shop. I didn't tell her what I was looking for, but it wasn't hard for her to guess. We'd watched *Monty Python and the Holy Grail* when we were kids, sharing a secret smile when the convent girls begged Galahad to spank them. And we'd played sadistic games, blackmailing each other into being a slave for a day or taking a hard slap on the inner thigh instead of being tattled on. She knew which way I was bent. And while we'd never explicitly discussed it, I knew she was bent the same way.

When we were little we used to act out stories. Of central importance to every scene was which one of us got to be 'poor'. That was our term for it. As in 'You poor thing!' It's the kind of argument only kinky children can have: 'No, it's my turn to be poor! You got to be poor last time!' Being poor covered anything from getting captured and tied up to being spanked. School scenes were always a favourite.

'If you're looking for spanking porn,' Jessie said without blushing, 'you need to meet my new boyfriend, Steve. He's got tons of CP mags and videos.'

'CP?'

'Corporal punishment.'

Spanking. Corporal punishment. Just hearing the words turned my knees to water. I couldn't even *say* them! I blushed furiously and tried to be offhand.

'Oh, yeah. Sure. Whatever.'

The first spanking video Steve showed me was called *Punishment PT*. It was awful. The dialogue was feeble and the premise was ludicrous. But it was a spanking video and that's what counted. Two English schoolgirls went across their gym master's knee for a hard bare-bottom spanking. It was *punishment*. It was *real*. I had never been so turned on in my life.

I was hooked, and Steve became my supplier. He plundered his archive, generously copying movies for me. I stayed up all night watching them, replaying again and again the bits that really made me hot. I had a TV in my room and I bought a special extension cable for my headphones. That way I could lie in bed at night and indulge myself without my parents wondering what all the smacking was.

I liked the English ones best. In my favourite, *College Classics 2*, a schoolgirl had to touch her toes for a dose of the cane from the headmaster. I must have watched that scene a thousand times. I was distraught when the tape finally broke.

The headmaster made her count aloud and say 'Thank you, sir' after each stroke. It became my most reliable masturbation aid. After the final stroke I'd rewind to the beginning of the sequence and play it again. And again. And again. When I finally came, I would picture myself in her position – bending over, gasping out the count, choking out a tearful 'Thank you, sir.' I still do.

Steve lent me magazines too. *Blushes. Janus. Uniform Girls.* *Blushes* was a treasure trove of politically incorrect fantasies featuring pretty young girls subject to discipline from strict older men. Not all of them with honourable intentions. There was one particular spread that I've never forgotten. A mortified choirgirl named Charlotte is positioned over a cushioned kneeler, her bottom raised up invitingly, to be caned by the vicar for messing around with a boy in the churchyard. In the second photoset, poor Charlotte and another girl are punished by both the vicar and the archdeacon.

If you're not a spanko you're probably wondering where sex fits into all this. It's hard to explain. For some, spanking is purely and overtly sexual. Even if it's punitive, it's really just extended foreplay, with sex the natural goal. For others – me among them – it's an act unto itself. The spanking *is* sex. It's *better* than sex. That's not to say I don't enjoy sex. I do, but only if I can pretend it's non-consensual. Unless it's a rape fantasy, it just doesn't turn me on. And even then it can't compete with the thrill of having my bottom smacked. But more of that later.

The pictures were exciting, but not all of the stories worked for me. That wasn't a problem; I simply made up my own to accompany the pictures. One thing I really disliked was any implication that the girl enjoyed being spanked. That spoiled it for me. Ironically, though I'm as kinky as they come, in all my fantasies I'm vanilla. The fact that in reality I'm wildly aroused and most definitely 'into' it is my little secret.

Best of all were the letters from readers. Men describing how they would deal with the neighbour's slutty daughter. Lovingly detailed accounts of the regimes they would impose on wayward girls if they owned their own reformatory. I imagined those stern older men watching *me* and writing letters discussing how they thought *I* should be punished.

But, much as I loved the magazines, I preferred the action of videos. I wanted to see the bottom reddening. I wanted to hear the smacks, the whoosh of the cane, the yelps and protests. And the English accents. I could think of nothing more exciting than being a rebellious American girl sent to a strict English boarding school.

Fetishists are obsessive collectors and I remember being blown away by the amount of material Steve had amassed. (My own collection puts it to shame now.) I was also surprised that he seemed so – well, *normal*. Here was an attractive college boy – not an obvious freak – with all this spanking porn. He wasn't a slavering pervert or a dirty old man. Of course it was hypocritical, but I'd never met any other spankos. I think most of us 'perverts' start off believing we're all alone in our desires.

One night Steve was visiting late. My parents had gone to bed and Steve, Jessie and I were watching a horror movie. Or, rather, we were pretending to watch it. Steve had brought me another fix of magazines and videos, but that wasn't all. When I saw the ping-pong paddle in his backpack, a shudder went through my whole body. I pressed my legs together, embarrassed at the instant wetness I felt.

'No way,' I said, but the tremor in my voice was unmistakable. It was the same tone I'd used as a little girl, daring the boys on the playground to chase me, catch me and tie me up. Oh, please, no, stop, anything but that . . .

'Stand up.'

My face burned and I looked at Steve in terror. I was frozen. The chair creaked behind me and, before I knew it, my sister had shoved me to my feet.

I was wearing a skimpy top and a short red tartan skirt that left little to the imagination. No one who knew me in school would have guessed I'd grow up to be such a shameless exhibitionist, but I was making up for lost time. Now I craved attention. I had worn the skirt just for Steve. To tease him.

He slid forwards until he was sitting on the edge of the sofa. The same one I'd been spanked behind by the king in my dream. Steve adjusted his glasses and looked at me, waiting.

I appealed to Jessie for help, but all she did was smile sadistically.

'Mom and Dad will hear,' I said in desperation.

With a soft laugh Jessie turned the volume up and the sound of screams and chainsaws filled the room.

Steve took my hand and pulled me firmly towards him. The inevitability sent a thrill through me and for a moment I was dizzy; I stumbled. Then he said it.

'Over my knee.'

I'd heard those words hundreds of times in movies and in my own head. But this time it was real. Blood pounded in my ears. I can't remember if he pulled me over or if I simply melted across his lap, but suddenly I found myself staring at the carpet. My skirt rode up and the air on my thighs made me feel exposed, vulnerable.

Steve rested his hand on my bottom. He gave me a few light pats over my skirt before Jessie told him to lift it.

'No!' I gasped.

I lay across his lap, trembling with fear and excitement. I strained to hear the creak of my parents' door over the noise from the TV, convinced that they would barge in any second.

When I felt Steve's hand on my panties I gave a little jump. They both laughed. I burned with shame. It would have been embarrassing enough with just Steve, but how could I endure it with my sister watching? We'd been spanked growing up, but never in front of each other.

The first smack sounded unbelievably loud and I couldn't hold back a yelp. It wasn't hard, but in my terror I thought it was agonising. I gritted my teeth and tried to keep quiet as he brought his hand down again and again on my bottom.

Every nerve in my body was wildly alive as I struggled and twisted on his lap, reaching back with my hands to protect my bottom. But Steve and I had seen the same movies; we knew what came next. He caught my wrists and pinned them in the small of my back, never breaking his cadence. I was helpless.

'That's nice and red,' Jessie said, making me cringe and hide behind my hair.

'Yes,' Steve agreed, 'but a naughty girl really only learns her lesson when her bottom is bare.'

My stomach plunged. He slipped his fingers into the elastic of my panties and tugged them down, exposing me. I squirmed, knowing my arousal was no secret to either of them. My panties were soaked.

I braced myself for another onslaught and when it came the noise was astonishing. So was the sting. It took me a minute to realise that he was using the ping-pong paddle. I'd forgotten all about it.

I howled as he delivered a fast volley of smacks. How could my parents not hear? The sound of a paddle is unmistakable. And my yelps and cries confirmed it. The TV could only mask so much.

I tried to block out my anxiety and submit to the moment. I had never felt so exposed. The feel of my panties twisted round my knees was both embarrassing and stimulating. And the heat blooming in my bottom was exquisite. It hurt, of course, but it was bearable. And every time Steve stopped to give me a rest I abandoned myself to the tingling and throbbing, drowning in sensations I couldn't process. I hated it. I loved it. I wanted it to stop. I didn't want it to end.

'Can't you do it harder than that?' Jessie asked suddenly.

I don't remember the conversation that followed because as soon as I realised where it was headed I felt faint. I stared at Jessie in horror, mouthing a frantic silent 'No!'

But they ignored my distress. Steve hauled me up off his lap and Jessie took his place. Mortified, I buried my face in my hands, moaning incoherent pleas.

Like all siblings, Jessie and I had had our violent fights and rough play. We each knew what the other could take. So I wasn't surprised when she slammed the paddle into my bottom with all the force she could muster. I choked back a scream and clutched the edge of the sofa as the pain washed over me. She hit me again and I made a strangled animal noise, forgetting all about my parents. The third one broke the paddle in two and they laughed as they allowed me to scramble up and adjust my clothes.

My bottom ached and throbbed, but the pain soon faded into a warm, pleasant glow. The skin felt raw and sunburned and I hissed as I pulled my panties back up. My face burned just as hotly; I couldn't face either of them.

Jessie and Steve split up a few weeks after that and I had to be satisfied with the movies he'd left me.

Unfortunately, about a year later I had another one of those misguided 'I can be normal' moments and destroyed the tapes. I regret it to this day; there were some real classics there.

Dear Niki,

I've been a fan of yours for a long time. However, I find thinking about you *making* a movie more exciting than watching the result. The thought of a woman willingly submitting to be whipped, caned, spanked, etc., is more truly exciting than the plot devices that require your character to submit to it through force.

J Jones, Canada

4. WEREWOLVES FROM THE EAST

'You have to see the new Lupus video,' said my friend Darcy. 'You'll love it.'

'What's it called?'

'*Stalin.*'

My boyfriend Cameron and I had already seen a few films by the Czech company Lupus Pictures (formerly Rigid East) and we were impressed by the quality of the productions. Each film opens with the animated image of a wolf raising its head to howl at the moon. The text below reads: 'We're wolves from East', which then changes to 'Werewolves from East'.

Spanking movies had come a long way, but many were still pretty amateurish. There was little attempt at plot and the dialogue was improvised. Cameras sat unmoving on tripods or lurched around like the handhelds in *The Blair Witch Project*. Girls being spanked stared fixedly in one direction, obviously watching themselves on off-screen monitors.

Lupus films were different. They were clearly made by professionals with professional equipment and an eye for authenticity. No other company had such elaborate plots, costumes and sets. The Lupus ethos was to transcend the genre by focusing on the context for the punishment. They wanted to show everything that happened before and after the climactic CP scene.

But Stalin? How could anyone make a spanking film about Stalin? I was intrigued. And Darcy was right; I loved it.

The setting is 1950s Communist Czechoslovakia. Lupus regular Kateřina Tetová plays the daughter of an executed political dissident. She and three friends have defaced a photograph of Stalin. Just a school prank to us, but a capital crime to the Party. The Communist commissar insists that the perpetrators be punished. Severely. After frightening the girls with talk of the brutal punishments administered in capitalistic schools, he decides that they should have a taste of them. He directs their form teacher to cane them.

A clever concept, well executed. But what I liked best was the form teacher, Alexandra Wolf. I'd seen her play the aloof and elegant mistress in a previous film. But here she was sympathetic. She wasn't sadistic or authoritarian; she was just following orders. And even while administering fifty hard strokes to each girl – except Kateřina, who got double – she managed to be compassionate. I'd always had a deep-seated resentment of female authority figures and all my fantasies were about men. Alexandra Wolf was the first female top I'd actually liked.

'I could imagine letting her cane me,' I confessed to Darcy.

Compassion is rare in Lupus films, which tend to favour uncompromising disciplinary situations. The movies may be a labour of love, but they're notorious for severe canings, most famously in the 'Headmaster's Study' series.

Set in the early 1900s, the series stars Pavel Šťastný, who also writes most of the screenplays. (Yes, screenplays. I did say they were pros.) An energetic fiftyish man with a shaved head and a booming voice, the irascible headmaster is a firm believer in the 'Austro-Hungarian rod'. And the Austro-Hungarian tradition is twenty-five strokes, not six. Misbehaving pupils find themselves strapped down over a specially designed whipping bench for canings that leave them bruised and sore.

It wasn't the severity of the punishments that appealed to me; it was the non-consensual context. Erotic spankings just don't do it for me; punishment is what pushes my buttons. Always has been. Consent has to exist in reality, but not in the fantasy. I don't need the *character* to consent; I'm watching a movie, not witnessing a crime.

Someone once wrote on a spanking forum that, by fetishising the suffering of others, we exploit and degrade the victims a second time. (I suspect he has a lot of issues with his own kink.) What such people don't understand is that I'm not eroticising the suffering of anyone but myself. I experience every scene, whether it's in a kinky or a mainstream film, through the eyes of the victim. My heart doesn't bleed for the predicaments of fictional characters; they're simply psychic costumes for me to put on and take off. Movies and books are projections of fantasy. A fantasy I can step into and play any part I want. And I'm *always* the victim.

Most BDSM and CP stories are cast from the 'victim's' point of view. And most tops prefer that perspective. While they fantasise about playing the dominant role in the scene, they want to know the girl's feelings and empathise with her suffering. Administering punishment imparts a charge, yes, but the real charge is in the intimate connection with the one surrendering to it. Think of the heroine in a horror film. The audience doesn't identify with the killer; they identify with the heroine.

But, playing devil's advocate, how do we know that what goes on behind the scenes really *is* consensual? Do the girls truly understand what they're getting into? Are they actually into it? Lupus was notorious enough in the early days to generate a few urban legends. People suggested that the Czech girls were poor and starving and would do anything for a crust of bread, even if it meant taking a savage caning. Were they drugged? How else could you get them to submit to such a thing? Most sinister of all was the suggestion that the girls might be trafficked and forced into it.

However, at the other end of the spectrum was another equally popular rumour – that it was all faked.

The early Rigid East films didn't have subtitles, which made them seem very grim indeed. I was certainly disturbed by the first one I ever saw, *The Catechist*. It was one of the early 'Headmaster's Study' episodes, very stark. Pavel Šťastný simply strapped a girl down to the punishment bench and caned her severely. Her distress upset me because I couldn't understand what she was yelling. Was she demanding to be let up? Or was she just acting? The fact that I couldn't tell made it hard for me to watch. I forced myself to stay until the end, however; I felt I owed it to her. And I needed to see her get up when it was all over.

An unscrupulous US-based company pirated a few Rigid East movies, relabelling them as 'Czech Brütal' (complete with heavy-metal umlaut) and hyping them as 'the strongest punishment videos ever filmed'. This lurid characterisation only reinforced the rumours.

The buzz was getting out of control. There were debates on the Internet spanking forums about whether Eastern European CP companies should be boycotted entirely. Since no one could be sure of the willingness of the participants or the ethics of the producers, there was some discomfort about enjoying the films.

No one in the English-speaking world knew anything about Lupus or what went on there. None of the Czech girls posted on the English forums. So there was no one to refute or confirm any of the rumours.

5. ALL DRESS MUST DOWN!

'*Záznam . . . Kamera . . . Akce!*'
    Brandishing the cane, Max bullies me into stripping off my school uniform.

'All dress must down!' he shouts.

My fingers shake so much I can barely manage the buttons. When I am down to my underwear, I turn away, ashamed. But he grabs me by the ear and drags me into the centre of the room, where I am forced to show him everything. He relishes my humiliation, saying obscene things to me in Czech that he knows I won't understand. I'm mortified, but I obey. I don't realise he's not the headmaster.

After he has his fill of ogling me, he pushes me down over the desk. With roaming hands, he positions me how he wants me – bottom out, legs apart, head up.

'Take it proudly,' he sneers in Czech.

Crying with fear and shame, I brace myself for what I think will be only six strokes. He raises the cane. By the time he is done I will have suffered 26. And after lunch I'll get another twelve from Alexandra Wolf.

Cameron and I thought it would be fun to spend Easter in Prague. We'd read about the *pomlázka* tradition and seen old postcards with laughing Slavic girls showing off their striped bottoms. The *pomlázka* (from *pomládit*, 'make younger') is a plaited whip made from pussywillow switches. According to Czech custom, it brings health and youth to girls whipped with it. Traditionally, on Easter Monday, the boys go carolling and whip any girls they can catch. Afterwards the girls reward them with Easter eggs, tying ribbons to the ends of the *pomlázky*. Girls who don't get whipped feel slighted. Surely it was an experience no spanko should be deprived of.

'Here's an idea,' I said. 'Maybe I can do a Lupus film while we're there!'

The website had hinted at a sequel to *Stalin*, set in the secret Communist prisons of the StB (secret police). My dark imagination ran wild and I began to spin my own fantasies about what might happen to a captured American spy in such a place.

I wasn't serious. But Cameron looked thoughtful. 'I wonder if you could,' he mused.

The idea began to obsess me. Could I really take that kind of punishment? Could I do it on camera? What if the rumours were true? Would I become a trafficked sex slave in Eastern Europe? Or worse – would I have to scream and struggle and pretend it hurt while they painted stripes on my bottom with makeup?

Finally, I emailed Lupus Pictures. Just to explore the possibility. I didn't actually think it would happen. I told myself they wouldn't have any interest in an American girl. After all, they presumably had their pick of starving Czech girls. But, to my surprise, they were very enthusiastic. And when producer Thomas Marco asked when they could schedule the shoot, I began to fret. My God, what had I let myself in for?

'Don't worry,' Cameron said. 'I won't abandon you in Prague. You're not going to the shoot alone.'

But what if they said no to a chaperone? I could understand why a film company wouldn't want boyfriends on the set. Besides, if Lupus had plans for me that involved me never going home, a boyfriend could make things difficult.

Before I could ask I got an email from Irena, the wardrobe and properties mistress, asking for my measurements. She said she was excited about the shoot and at the end of her email she said, 'Of course, your boyfriend is welcome too.' Of course. My fears about being abducted were beginning to fade.

Thomas said the script for *Stalin 2* wasn't ready yet, but he liked the idea of an exchange-student scenario. He sent me a synopsis and it was just my kind of scene: a 'fish out of water' story exploiting the language barrier.

We wrote back and forth over the next few days. I had just seen *The Nightmare*, the latest instalment in the 'Headmaster's Study' series. There was a zealous young Czech army officer in it, played by Maxmilian Schubert, the commissar from *Stalin*. He looked hot in his uniform (I'm a sucker for uniforms), but what I really liked was his Prussian-style heel-clicking and saluting. It appealed to my military fetish. I asked Thomas if Max could be the top in my story. He replied that I would be caned by two different tops and that Max could certainly be one of them.

'Two?' I gulped.

He sent me an English translation of the finished screenplay and I read it at once. First I would be caned by an impostor (Max) and then I would be caned by the real headmaster (Lars Moebius). I had never seen Lars in a film before. My nervousness grew. I'd seen Max in action, but Lars was a complete unknown.

In addition, the lengthy script was intimidating. It wasn't just a sketchy roleplay where we'd improvise the dialogue, but a thirty-page screenplay with scripted lines. I hadn't anticipated that. Practising my lines with Cameron felt unnatural and stilted, as I was used to improv. I was a roleplayer, not an actress. Was I out of my depth?

The days leading up to the Prague trip felt like the final days before an execution. I had bizarre dreams about what the shooting would be like. When I could sleep, that was. Cameron had to do a lot of reassuring, though part of him was enjoying my dread. I was sure I'd be enjoying it too – once it was over.

Then I got an email from Thomas headed 'change of plans'. My heart sank when I saw the subject line. They didn't want me after all.

'Lars Moebius is not available on those dates,' he wrote, 'so we changed his character.'

I was going to be caned by Alexandra Wolf.

6. EXCHANGE STUDENT

The year is 1938. A snappily dressed man is nosing around in a headmaster's office when an English girl enters with a note from her teacher. According to the note, she's been fighting with her schoolmates and is to be punished. The man looks her over, getting ideas. He smiles.

After taking advantage of his opportunity to strip her and cane her, he stands her against the wall and slips out. A few moments later, a woman arrives and asks what the girl is doing there. The girl tells her that the headmaster just caned her. Confused, the woman explains that the headmaster is out of town. Then she reads the note. She informs the girl that she is the Deputy Headmistress and will punish her in place of the headmaster. The girl insists that she's already been punished, but the Deputy Headmistress won't hear it. Defeated, the girl fetches the cane again and bares her bottom for another caning. Afterwards the secretary comes in, startled to see what's going on. She asks what happened to the insurance agent who was waiting there. At last the Deputy Headmistress understands.

When the girl has regained her composure, the Deputy Headmistress asks her why she was fighting and the girl breaks down and confides the awful story. She's new to the country and the Czech girls have been bullying her. Today they started a fight with her and, when the teacher broke it up, the other girls claimed she'd started it. So he sent the English girl to be punished.

The culprits are sent for and each girl takes forty hard strokes while the English girl watches, grinning triumphantly. The movie ends with the Deputy Headmistress rejoicing in her success at restoring international peace, speaking appreciatively of England, the true ally of Czechoslovakia, currently fighting in Munich for 'peace in our time'.

The credits roll to the sound of jackboots and a Czech news report about Chamberlain's infamous appeasement of Hitler.

On the day set for the rehearsal Lupus sent a cab to fetch us from our hotel in central Prague. There was a bit of comedy when we got to the drab suburban office block that housed the studio, as the entrance was padlocked. I wandered round to another entrance, where a woman at the door shouted something at me in Czech. At the time my Czech didn't consist of much more than 'please', 'thank you' and 'Where's the loo?' I offered her Thomas's and Irena's names and she shook her head.

With a sense of disappointment and relief I shrugged. 'I guess it's the wrong address,' I told Cameron. But then I mentioned 'Lupus' and understanding dawned in her face. She rolled her eyes and yelled something up the stairs, at which point a cheerful young brunette – Irena – came running down to greet us. There was no backing out now.

Irena led us into a nondescript office suite behind a door in a glass-and-plastic screen. I looked around in disbelief. *This* was where all those poor girls were beaten and tortured? It was so normal it was surreal. Fair enough; Prague's the hometown of Kafka, after all.

All the Lupus stars were there. I met Alexandra Wolf and headmaster Pavel Šťastný. Maxmilian Schubert clicked his heels for me, making me blush. I didn't know anyone and yet I knew everyone. Even the director, Zbyšek Podhajský, had been in a few videos.

Kateřina Tetová was there too, though she wasn't going to be in the film. She had starred in several Lupus productions since *Stalin* and had many adoring fans in the west. They would be so envious to know that I had met her. I couldn't wait to tell them that she was even lovelier in person. But I also knew they would be crushed to learn that she wasn't available; she was Max's girlfriend.

After the dizzying round of introductions, Michal Valášek, the executive producer, took me into the back room to go over the contract. He's a long-haired techie who plays some of the quirkier Lupus roles.

Stashed in a corner of his office was the whipping bench from the headmaster's study. I was surprised how small it was. But, then, everything is larger than life on the screen. I couldn't resist bending over it for Cameron to smack me over my jeans.

Signing the contract was an adventure. There was no English version, so poor Michal had to go through the eight-page document line by line and translate. It's an interesting question whether a contract in a language I don't speak is valid or not. Sort of like a confession signed in a foreign jail. Cameron thought my status as a *kaskadérka* (stuntgirl) was a stroke of genius. With an unsteady hand I signed away my fate.

Max was having fun with the broken English lines he had to say ('You did make big mistake!' 'All dress must down!' 'I vill beat you!'), so it was hard to be completely serious during the rehearsal. At first the dialogue felt awkward; however, once I got into the flow of doing each scene piece by piece it began to sound more natural. But Zbyšek told me I wasn't speaking loudly enough. It's a challenge to be meek and frightened and yet loud enough to be heard. It isn't a problem in roleplay.

I was very intimidated by Pavel Šťastný until he sashayed in wearing a wig and putting on a flamboyant show. After that I found it hard to be afraid of him. He helped me with my Czech lines and tried to teach me how to pronounce the impossible ř letter. It's a sound unique to Czech – a rolled R and a French J ('zh') said together. To this day I still can't do it.

The rehearsal reminded me of my high-school drama days, where there was more clowning around than serious acting. But we mapped out the scenes for the next day and the director seemed happy. Cameron and I hung around chatting until our cab came to take us back to the hotel. We were scheduled to be at the studio again early the next morning. I didn't know if I'd be able to sleep.

I'd been lying awake for about an hour when the alarm went off at six a.m. I didn't feel at all well. I felt cold and clammy and my stomach was doing gymnastics.

It wasn't just the pain I was afraid of. The shoot would preserve my image forever, on film and across the Internet. The UK has the harshest censorship in Europe: it's illegal to sell CP videos, and

HM Customs often confiscates material that is perfectly legal in the rest of the continent. Could they arrest me for participating? I didn't know, but I could hardly ask. And what would my parents think? What had I got myself into?

All at once I couldn't breathe. My stomach lurched and I just made it to the bathroom, falling to my knees in front of the toilet. It wasn't pretty.

I emerged at last, pale, shaky and embarrassed. But I felt immensely better. Cameron made me a cup of tea (is that the English solution to everything?) and I was back to normal by the time I'd drunk it.

I couldn't believe I'd been so freaked out. I'd been fantasising about the shoot for weeks. There was no way I would deprive myself of an experience like this. I couldn't live in my parents' looming shadow all my life and I would never forgive myself if I chickened out now.

The panic attack was over and I was ready for the shoot. Ready to experience first-hand either a fake caning or abuse by savage wolves.

They were serving breakfast when we arrived, but I couldn't eat. Now that I was back in the studio, my anxiety was returning. Fortunately, there was nothing left in my system for it to play havoc with.

The actual shooting wasn't due to start for several hours, but they'd wanted me there early. It was what I'd always heard about making movies in Hollywood – that it was 90 per cent waiting. Punishments are always worse when they're delayed. I felt like a girl who'd been sent to see the headmaster only to be told to come back later. Hours later.

The professionalism of the team really impressed me. In addition to the director, producer, script supervisor, makeup artist, properties and wardrobe mistress, caterer, cameramen, boom operator, still photographer, actors and (ahem) stuntgirls, there were people on hand to offer us refreshments, comfort or anything else we needed. This was not a couple of pornographers making dirty pictures in a basement, nor was it a band of misogynists taking advantage of girls who couldn't say no. This was a real film crew working on a real film. The tech guys were all professional camera and sound men, hired for their expertise. Not kinky themselves, they nonetheless took their job seriously and worked as diligently as they would have on any mainstream project.

It was nearly one o'clock and at last it was time to start shooting. This was an unusual movie for Lupus because the first punishment scene comes right at the beginning. They've been known to spend an hour of screen time on plot development before any actual punishment. It was also unusual because they had never made an English-language film before and most of this one was in English. They were counting on me, a complete unknown, not only to carry the film, but also to attract international attention and English-speaking fans. It was a huge responsibility.

Throughout the morning, Irena had been like a mother hen, checking on me often and trying to get me to eat. I reassured her I was fine, explaining that I was just nervous. She made me promise her I'd eat something once the scary part was over.

To my surprise, Zbyšek said he wasn't going to shoot the caning all in one go. He explained the sequence: Max would give me one hard stroke to intimidate me into stripping off. Then he'd give me a formal six of the best that I would count. (My character thinks that's all she's going to get.) But then he'd haul me back over the desk, explaining that the Czech tradition was 25 strokes, and he'd give me the rest in two batches. Zbyšek was very careful framing and setting up for the first stroke because it couldn't be reshot once I was marked. By this point I was paralysed with fear. I was about to get what I was sure would be the hardest caning of my life.

I lay over the desk, frightened and humiliated, looking worriedly at Max and insisting that it wouldn't be proper to undress in front of him. (It's 1938, after all.)

'So we understand each other,' he growled at me in Czech, raising the cane. I heard the swoosh and the crack of the impact, but, to my amazement, I hardly felt it at all! I was completely lost in the moment and the pressure of so many people watching. It was a feeling I would come to know very well. I reacted as I was supposed to, but I was truly *acting*.

Stripping for the camera was a nerve-racking experience. But my fear heightened the erotic thrill. I was buzzing with an inner intensity as I surrendered to Max's humiliation of an innocent girl. I didn't have to be bold and confident, displaying my charms with no trace of shame. My character was mortified, so *I* was mortified.

My embarrassment over being the only one naked in a room of fully clothed people faded soon enough, though; I had another six strokes coming. These were the ones I was meant to count. And again, I barely felt them. Perhaps it was fake after all. Was Max even hitting me? Zbyšek yelled 'Cut!' and Thomas came running over to check on me.

'I'm fine,' I said, baffled to find that I was. I felt a little tender, but it was nothing like I'd expected, nothing like the films I'd seen. Had those girls all just been overreacting?

I rejected that thought instantly once the final strokes began. Max ramped it up and Cameron told me afterwards that he was using full arm strokes, which is hard to do accurately. My regular play partners always gave me precisely aimed strokes that landed on my bottom and didn't wrap, but Max caned me with uneven diagonal strokes, landing the cane tip on my right thigh. Cameron said it was very hard to watch. Fortunately, Kateřina was there to comfort him during the worst moments.

By this time I was feeling every stroke acutely. And crying. Yes, *this* was what I had been expecting. I was in so much pain that I had no idea how many strokes I'd taken. I couldn't have said whether it was five or fifty. It was just a haze of pain.

I've never considered myself to be a masochist. I cringe and wince when I watch CP films, insisting, 'I could never take that!' But it's not a matter of 'what I can take'; to live my fantasies I have no choice *but* to take it. The feeling of being out of control is extremely heady. And, while I enjoy the fantasy, halfway into the reality I start to believe I'm vanilla. Afterwards, of course, I bask in the glow of the subsiding pain and marvel at what I've endured. I can't enjoy it unless I don't enjoy it.

When the caning finally stopped I lay there sobbing over the desk for several seconds. The room was silent but for my sobs. It was eerie. I felt like I was the only person in the world.

Then Zbyšek yelled 'Cut!' and everyone applauded. Thomas rushed over to ask if I was OK and I managed a sniffly smile and told him I was fine. He said I was doing great and asked if I was ready to finish the caning. I gasped. I hadn't realised it wasn't over yet.

The next strokes were even worse and I clung to the desk as they sliced into my bottom one by one. And my right thigh. Again, I had no idea how many strokes it was, though I knew I was near the end. And when it was finally over, I cried in silence again. It was such a strange place to be. I was utterly alone with my pain and yet I didn't feel isolated. There was a roomful of people watching me and I was perfectly safe. I had the feeling of jumping from a height with the total certainty that someone would catch me. A sense of euphoria began to build and I felt suddenly lighter. Through a fog I heard 'Cut!' and some muted applause. Then a pair of arms encircled me and I realised it was Cameron.

Some submissives can have orgasms from intense whippings. I've always envied them. While I didn't have a physical orgasm, this was the emotional equivalent. It was a level of exhilaration I had never experienced before and I didn't want it to end. There's a point where the pain becomes something else. Not pleasure exactly, but something between the two extremes of feeling. Something *more* than the two. It's indefinable. I was flying.

If it had been a roleplay I would have curled up in Cameron's arms for as long as it took to drift back to reality. But you don't have that luxury when you're shooting. We had to finish the scene before the marks started to fade.

Exchange Student has its comedic moments and one of the funniest scenes was unintentional. Under the school blazer I wore a white shirt and, under that, a white undershirt – no modern bra for the authenticity fetishists at Lupus. When Max made me strip, I was off to one side when I took off my blazer, shirt and tie. Then he pulled me to the centre of the room to take off my skirt, knickers and undershirt. When he told me to get dressed after the caning he reached down and handed me the nearest thing, which was my shirt. I was still crying and my hands were shaking visibly as I buttoned it. Halfway through I realised I didn't have my undershirt. But Max had already moved the clothes, so the continuity person said they couldn't reshoot it. Zbyšek cut and there was some discussion.

Finally, Max suggested something in Czech and I heard the word 'fetish'. Everyone burst out laughing. I looked over at Max and he demonstrated for me: he picked up my undershirt, sniffed it and put it in his pocket! So we shot the rest of the scene and the insurance agent made off with his victim's undershirt. It was a wonderfully pervy touch.

After Max stood me facing the wall and sneaked off, we broke for lunch. I got a bone-crushing bear hug from him and then another from Cameron. I ate my roast chicken standing up.

A caning hurts when it's given and it keeps on hurting for a long time afterwards. You don't forget it in a hurry – as any English schoolboy knows. So an hour later, my bottom was still throbbing and I couldn't sit comfortably. And it was time for my second caning. Now I was really starting to question my sanity.

Alexandra Wolf is a very skilled and experienced domme. I was to get twelve strokes from her on top of my twenty-six from Max. I raised my skirt, lowered my knickers and resumed my place over the desk. As she raised the cane, I took a deep breath.

It was hard, but nowhere near as hard as what Max had given me. And it was far more accurate. But on my already sore bottom it hurt plenty. Still, I diligently counted each stroke and thanked her. I had hoped they'd make me do it in Czech but, as I was playing the good little English girl, Zbyšek thought it was more appropriate to have me count in English.

I didn't experience the same exhilaration this time. I think I'd spent all my endorphins on the first caning. But I had the same sense of accomplishment. And the marks to show for it. Now I could relax. My two 'bullies' had just arrived and it would soon be their turn to bend over the desk for a dose of the cane.

Our Prague guidebook had said that the older generation wouldn't speak English, but that the younger generation would. The reverse was the case. The girls and I were limited to communicating mostly through smiles and sign language. Poor Zbyšek had to speak two languages all day, which made his job twice as hard.

I was amazed by Denisa Petráková, who played one of the bullies. A first-timer, the little blonde bravely took forty hard full-arm strokes from Alexandra, sobbing the whole time. I was wincing at every stroke, though I was meant to look smug and triumphant. Eva Šulistová took her forty strokes more stoically, but she'd been in several previous films.

As with me, there was a pause after every ten to fifteen strokes to check that the girls were OK. The crew couldn't have been more concerned for our safety. Both girls survived and it wasn't long before they were laughing and joking. The 'after' shots on the Lupus website show the three of us smiling, laughing and posing for silly pictures sporting vivid tramlines. Abused? Us?

The shoot was exhausting, but I didn't want it to end. In the beginning it was hard to tune out the cameras and the technical distractions, but once I was actually in the scene I could lose myself in the character. The experience blurred the line between reality and fantasy many times and those are moments I treasure.

It was easy for me to be the unfortunate English exchange student because I truly didn't understand what was being said around me, so, when I was meant to feel alienated, I did.

The next day Cameron and I went to Karlštejn Castle southwest of Prague – a most uncomfortable train ride on the hard seats. But even though I enjoyed the trip I was a little low in spirits. It was over. A fantastic party had ended and I was coming down from an incredible high. All I could think was: when can I do it again?

Hey, no one ever accused me of being normal.

I find it difficult to believe that Niki Flynn has any credibility in her posts. Maybe she is for real, but more likely she is doing a good PR job for Lupus/Rigid East, who produce films of extreme violence towards women.

Marvin, UK

7. AN AMERICAN WEREWOLF IN PRAGUE

It was a big decision, making the leap from amateur enthusiast to professional victim. You have to be prepared for immortality. Fame and popularity fade, of course, but, if you suddenly get religion one day, you can't just obliterate your work. Your face and body are all over the Net and on thousands of strange computers. Long after you've retired or died.

Exchange Student was in postproduction and I needed a stage name for the film credits. Some models have fanciful names like Venus or Genesis, but those names don't work in a school setting. I've always found the English practice of addressing pupils by their surnames inexplicably erotic. Uniforms and surnames – it's so militaristic. The name had to be believable.

Czech is merciless. Surnames like 'Pospíšilová' and 'Myšičková' don't trip easily from Western tongues. Those consonants and diacriticals take no prisoners.

By the way, if you think those are hard, here's an actual Czech tongue-twister: '*Strč prst skrz krk*' (stick your finger through your throat). Actually, that one's not so bad. Remember the unpronounceable ř? The really evil one is '*Třistatřiatřicet stříbrných křepelek přeletělo přes třistatřiatřicet stříbrných střech*' (333 silver quails flew over 333 silver roofs).

I wanted a Czech-friendly stage name, but one that would be easy for non-Czechs as well. I chose 'Nicki' – a tribute to Nicki

Brand in *Videodrome* – and I Easternised the spelling by dropping the 'c'. I decided I wanted an Irish surname and 'Niki Flynn' sounded spunky and adventurous. Especially as the combination rhymed with 'Mickey Finn'. I never anticipated such confusion, though; I've seen every possible spelling of Niki.

When I joined Internet spanking forums, I didn't want to say where I really lived, so in my profiles I listed 'Prague' as my location. That caused confusion too and I got charming notes from people complimenting me on my English. I appreciated the compliment, since my first language isn't English; it's American.

Thomas asked me as a favour to try and dispel the myth about starving, drugged and trafficked girls. He didn't care about the rumours that the canings were faked; he just wanted people to know they weren't abusing or exploiting disadvantaged girls.

I wrote an account of my experience under the title 'West Meets East', which Lupus published on their website. I also posted on the spanking forums, doing what I could to clear up the misconceptions. I felt like a reporter who'd gone undercover to discover the truth behind the urban legends. And while my initial purpose in posting had been only to debunk the Lupus rumours, I soon succumbed to the lure of daily spanking chat and became a regular participant.

Most of the members were friendly and welcoming and many were interested in hearing about the shoot. I loved reliving the experience, so I was happy to talk about it. What I wasn't prepared for were the attacks. More than one person accused me of being a PR whore for Lupus, as though I got rake-offs for every film they sold.

There's a well-known saying in kinky circles: a pervert is anyone kinkier than I am. The One True Way spankos know exactly what they like; anything outside those boundaries is depraved. They insisted that my fantasies were sick and that Lupus films promoted violence towards women. It's the same argument people have levelled against horror films for years. They assume that all viewers identify with the sadist/killer/rapist, ignoring the thousands of masochists who identify with the victim/heroine. Any BDSM survey will tell you that submissive males are the majority and there are plenty of films to accommodate their interests. But no one worries about films promoting violence towards men.

There's a Ph.D. thesis in there somewhere, I'm sure.

I spent hours arguing on the controversial threads. The violence accusation was always guaranteed to stir me up. But it wasn't the most frustrating one. Despite my accounts to the contrary, loads of people simply refused to believe the punishment was real. They were certain it was all faked and they didn't want to be confused with the facts. Maddening! A production crew with a budget like *Lord of the Rings* might be able to fake a caning with special effects and makeup, but who in their right mind would bother when there are plenty of us willing to do it for real? Marks develop *after* a stroke lands. So not only would you have to create the initial marks, for each successive stroke you'd have to enhance the mark from the previous stroke to keep the developing bruises and stripes consistent. That would mean cutting after every single stroke. It would take days of shooting and weeks of postproduction. The cost would be astronomical.

One man wrote to console me. He was a professional stuntman for mainstream movies and TV shows and he said he had the exact same problem. People would scoff at a death-defying leap from a burning building and say, 'Oh, that's obviously just a mannequin.' It was infuriating for him. But it made me feel a little better. At least I wasn't risking my *life*.

'But you don't see the cane land every time. The camera cuts away to the girl's face.'

Not nearly enough for some, who prefer to see the emotions in the girl's face. If you *never* saw the cane land, I could understand the scepticism. But, as it is, half the time you see the face and half the time you see the bottom. It's a nice balance.

'Of course you're going to defend them. They're paying you, aren't they?'

Sigh. They *paid* me for my role in the film. But it was a fixed fee; the working relationship ended there. No one was paying me to play on the forums and talk about the fun I'd had shooting a movie. No one needed to.

But the most baffling accusation was that I wasn't really into spanking at all. I was only in it for the money. There was nothing to do but laugh at that. I couldn't imagine what kind of money they thought I made. It actually barely covered my travel expenses. If I wasn't into spanking, surely I could find easier and less painful ways to earn that pittance than by getting beaten in the Czech Republic!

One man I corresponded with was surprised to learn that I

wasn't rich. He'd assumed spanking models got paid A-list Hollywood salaries and lived like movie stars. If only!

For the record, it's a professional wage. It's certainly not going to make me rich. And considering that it often takes several weeks to heal fully from a shoot, it's not something I can do more than once or maybe twice a month. My normal rate is £600 a day for moderate severity – more if I'm going to be marked for more than a week and unable to work. The most I've ever been paid for a single shoot is €1200. (That's about $1500 or £800.) Even if I could guarantee one shoot a month at that rate, it would barely cover my rent.

In the eye of this teacup storm I got an email from David Pierson. He maintains spreview.net, a website that provides reviews of spanking videos together with industry news and interviews with spanking models. He said he'd always admired Lupus's work and was interested in hearing about their operation. He wanted me to do an interview.

I said I'd be happy to, but I was leery of sharing too much personal information, as I'd been stalked in the past. He assured me that I didn't have to say anything I didn't want to.

One of the things he said he had to ask was whether I'd been spanked as a child. Well, I had, but I didn't really want to talk about it; the memories aren't erotic. Nor did I feel comfortable publishing any real details about my childhood. I assumed people would be reading the interview mainly for titillation, so I decided to make it just as titillating for me.

I created a fantasy background. I said I grew up in a large Irish Catholic family in Boston. (I am part Irish, but I was raised by heathens and I've never even been to Boston.) Instead of my one kinky sister I claimed to have several brothers. I've always had a thing for brother/sister scenes, so I said I'd often been punished by my oldest brother after my father walked out. Hey, it's a fantasy business and I thought it only fair that I be allowed my fantasies too.

Jessie loved that I made her a brother in the interview. Kink-wise, she's a gay man in a woman's body. She asked if she could stay a brother in this memoir as well. But, while I'm comfortable changing names to protect people's privacy, I wanted to come clean here about my fictional family life. Sorry, sis!

The interview made me feel like a celebrity. I got lots of positive feedback, with people asking when *Exchange Student* would be out. And I figured that was that. A few viewers asked me when I would be doing more CP film work, but I told them it was a one-off. I'd lived my fantasy on film and, to quote David, 'gone down in the annals of spanking cinema history as the first girl from the west to take a caning from the infamous Werewolves from the East'. That was something to be proud of.

Accuracy is more important to me than severity. If the stripes are evenly distributed, and leave vivid red lines only on the lower half of the buttocks and not on the hips, that is the look I like.

No matter the implement, I always appreciate a decorous result, and it's more than just aesthetics. When the ordeal is over and done, the lesson clearly imprinted for what may be many days ahead, it should look like a punishment given very thoughtfully and deliberately, not wild and spontaneous as if in a fit of anger. It suggests to me a very calculated method of discipline, and that the receiver was under the rigid control of the administrator. It adds to the ritualism.

xoxoxo,

Eric, California

8. CRIME AND PUNISHMENT

'No, please!'
'Česky!'
'Ne, prosím!'

I have no idea how many times the cane has slashed into my bottom. I'm in so much pain I'm barely able to draw breath to cry out, let alone translate my hysterical pleas into Czech. At least I don't have to worry about staying in position. The straps around my arms, legs and waist ensure that I will take every stroke.

When the caning is finally over I lie limp across the bench, sobbing. The other three girls release me and I slump to my knees on the floor. But the headmaster isn't finished with me yet.

'Miss Čermaková,' he says in Czech as he looms over me. 'You have exploited and defiled the very essence of womanhood. You are a disgrace to your sex and you don't deserve to be seen as a creature of glamour and beauty.'

My face streaming with tears, I raise my head in confusion. And I scream when I see what he intends.

The other girls hold me in position as he brandishes the scissors. He seizes my hair, yanking my head up roughly. I hear a snip and a lock of my hair falls to the floor in front of me. I struggle, but I am no match for three girls bent on retribution. The headmaster forces my head up again, making me cry out. The scissor blades are dull and the pain is terrible as he saws through my glossy curls. With every cut he strips me of my dignity, my femininity, my vanity. The wiles I used to corrupt and manipulate the girls who hold me still for him. No mercy for the gangster's daughter.

Defeated, I can only watch helplessly as wisps of hair drift to the floor around me. And when the deed is done, my hands flutter hesitantly to my scalp, feeling the short spiky hair that is left. I cover my head as the shame overwhelms me and I sink to the floor, crushed, humiliated, beaten.

'Lupus is going to do *what*?'

That was the reaction I got from most of my friends when I told them about my next project.

'Cut off my hair,' I explained patiently. 'Look, I've had short hair before. And it will grow back.'

'Niki, have you ever been told that you're a weird little shit?'

I smiled. 'All my life.'

It's the early 1900s. The Austro-Hungarian Empire. Crime has reared its ugly head at the prestigious St Thomas's School for Girls. The police raid a pornographic photography studio and open fire, killing both the photographer and his model. The only clue left behind is a photo album. The police commissioner shows the album to Headmaster Šťastný and asks him if he recognises any of the girls. He does, but he denies it. When he confronts the three students with the photos, they confess: the modelling sessions were arranged by Elisabeth Čermaková, a Czech-American student. She also happens to be the daughter of a notorious American gangster.

Mr Šťastný is despondent. This will ruin him. He confides in a youthful Sigmund Freud, who propounds absurd sexual theories about father figures, phallic canes and the erotic implications of punishment. In desperation, the headmaster explains that he needs to get rid of Čermaková. Preferably without killing her. That's the easy part, Freud tells him. The headmaster must undertake a psychic castration – strip her of her power. Take away her femininity.

The next day the headmaster has the three 'models' report to his study. Since they were willing to pose naked in the photographs, they can be naked for their punishment. Each girl spends a long painful time strapped down over the bench as he administers forty strokes with the cane. Now it is time to confront the real culprit.

Čermaková is defiant; however, when threatened with the police, she confesses the truth. The photographer was her boyfriend and she procured the girls for him so the two of them could sell the photos and earn passage back to America. Sending her to America is fine with Mr Šťastný, but she's not going anywhere until she's paid for her sins. When she refuses to undress he has the three other girls tear her clothes off and strap her to the bench. Since Čermaková's crime was the worst, she gets ten extra strokes. Then, as a final humiliation, he cuts her hair. She won't be showing her face in public any time soon.

I was excited about getting to play the villain, but I was intimidated by the dialogue. This time, nearly all my lines were in Czech. While my language skills had improved since the first shoot, I still knew only a few useful words and phrases. I had to learn my lines phonetically.

While the dialogue was a challenge, it wasn't as scary as the prospect of a caning from Pavel Šťastný. The headmaster's severity was legendary among Lupus fans.

The cane is truly unique. Let me try to describe it. A typical school cane is a crook-handled length of flexible rattan three feet long but only a quarter of an inch thick. Perhaps a little more. Think of it as a whip made of wood. It twists in the air like a living thing and it takes a lot of skill to wield it properly. A lot of practice, too.

When the stroke lands you feel the impact, but there's a split-second delay before you actually feel any pain. Then the thin stripe starts to burn. And burn. And burn. Like a wave the pain swells and crests while you surf it, going where it takes you. By the time it peaks it's time for another stroke.

Timing is important and a skilled caner knows just how long to wait and when to strike again. The next stroke hurts even more and the next hurts even more than that. By this time, pain is your whole world and the surging waves threaten to pull you under. You have to stay on top. It's about survival and triumph. The reward at the end is worth it.

I love the cane and I hate it just as passionately. It *hurts*.

The single most common question people ask me is how I can take it. T.E. Lawrence put it best: the trick is not *minding* that it hurts.

* * *

Lupus scheduled the shoot to coincide with the premiere of *Exchange Student*. For each film they hire a kink-friendly venue for a private party where they have a screening for their friends. It was great to see everyone again. In the English-speaking world I had become a sort of ambassador for Lupus Pictures, for which they were very grateful.

Seeing myself on film was strange enough, but seeing myself *caned* on film was positively surreal. It looked much worse than it had felt at the time. It was so intense I almost couldn't watch. Cameron squeezed my hand reassuringly as the hardest strokes fell. He said afterwards that watching the movie was almost as hard for him as watching the actual caning.

I also learned what all actors learn when they see themselves on film for the first time. The camera *does* add ten pounds and they'll always use the worst take. Watching yourself on film is a special kind of torment; you see every flaw and second-guess every line delivery. Naturally, you're your own harshest critic and much of what seems obvious to you goes unnoticed by everyone else. The adult industry offers even more cause for embarrassment. Before *Exchange Student*, no one but my gynaecologist had ever seen me at such close range. I tried not to think about that too much.

Back once more at the familiar studio, I met the three girls who would be my co-stars. They were all newbies, and again didn't speak much English. When I asked Michal how they found the girls he explained that Lupus was mostly a core group of friends in the Czech BDSM scene. Some of the girls were kinky friends of theirs and others came from a local acting agency. My jaw dropped. An acting agency?

He went on to say that the girls came in for an audition, where they saw photographs and clips from the movies. Then they were given a few strokes of the cane so they could decide whether it was something they were prepared to do. They often said it was no worse than they'd had from their parents at home.

The first scene was the shootout at the photography studio. Since the photographer was supposed to be American, they needed someone who could do an American accent. Cameron's British, but I did my best as dialect coach.

Petr Podhajský played the photographer while Cameron dubbed his voice. It was hard not to crack up at the things he had to say as the sleazy pornographer. 'Come on, baby,' he breathed into the microphone, sounding like an obscene phone caller. 'Let's see those little tits. Now show me what you've got between your legs. That's it, yeah, they'll love you in America, baby.'

We were both impressed by the attention to period detail. There was an antique gramophone in the corner, which Petr wound up and played. And when he took pictures of the model, he used an actual magnesium flash with powder in a cup. Neither of us had ever seen one used before.

The police burst into the room and Petr pulled a gun, grabbing the model to use as a hostage. A deafening gunfight ensued and we were relieved to discover that there are some things that Lupus does fake. Neither Petr nor the model was actually shot, though the bloodstains on the walls and floor were very convincing.

I spent most of the next day with my hair in oversize curlers. Magda, the makeup artist, gave me a big fancy hairstyle befitting an arrogant gangster's daughter. I barely recognised myself. I was nervous, but very excited as well. This was something that had never been done in a CP film before and it was a long-standing fantasy of mine. The ultimate humiliation.

My one big worry was that viewers would think it was a wig. And why wouldn't they? Surely no girl would be crazy enough to have her hair shorn just for a kinky movie. In fact, Pavel told me he'd been wanting to do a forced haircut for ages, but that none of the Czech girls would do it. Caning was fine, but no one was going to touch their hair! Strike another blow for that 'They're so desperate they'll do anything' argument.

If I'd thought it was strange seeing myself caned on film, it was even stranger being in the headmaster's study. The setting was so familiar. I'd seen all the videos in the series and I had fantasised about being caned over the whipping bench. The same bench I had so playfully bent over in the office back in the spring. It didn't seem so small now. Now it was centre stage and in just a few hours I would be suffering over it. It was like stepping through a movie screen and onto the set.

It's fascinating to watch a girl take her first-ever caning. The first girl, Klára, didn't react to the first stroke right away. She looked bewildered and uncertain what to expect. But by the second stroke she was beginning to appreciate its sting. Cameron and I watched, wide-eyed, as Pavel marked her pale skin with bright-red stripes. She struggled against the restraints, howling in pain. For some reason it always looks worse when someone else is getting it. And as Pavel brought the whippy rattan down on her bottom over and over again I reminded myself that I would be getting the same, plus an extra ten strokes.

After the agreed first fifteen strokes, Pavel raised the cane and held his position until Zbyšek yelled, 'Cut!' Thomas rushed over to Klára to make sure she was OK. She was visibly shaken and crying, but she said she was fine. The cameras rolled again and she took another fifteen. There was a final break and then the last ten strokes, which were the hardest of all.

But poor Klára's ordeal wasn't over yet. She had to stand against the wall with her hands on her head, her bottom on display, while the next girl had her turn over the bench. Then both girls stood there in disgrace, sniffling, while the last one took her forty strokes.

Cameron and I felt drained after watching the punishments. All three girls got a round of applause and then it was time for lunch, which, naturally, I couldn't eat. I'd been sick that morning, just as on the morning of my first shoot. Apparently it was my body's way of coping with the anxiety. Not very glamorous. Despite Irena's protests, I said I was on hunger strike until after my caning.

Pavel grinned at me. We'd been exchanging emails in a combination of fractured English and Czech since the first shoot. He knew how much I'd been dreaming about a visit to the headmaster's study and he knew how much I wanted to push myself.

Outside in the corridor the three girls were lying on their stomachs with damp towels over their bottoms. They had tear-stained faces, but were otherwise happily chatting to each other and comparing notes on the experience.

Pavel and I had a lengthy scene before my stripping and caning. While I had learned all my lines phonetically, I had an English translation of the script to tell me what I was saying. Czech is a highly complex language, but at least it has consistent pronunciation rules. Learning the sounds wasn't as difficult as learning which words and syllables to inflect to make the dialogue sound natural. It's not enough just to tell me that 'Co mohu já udělat pro soud dělat neřešit?' means 'What do I have to do to keep the authorities from getting involved?' I had to ask Zbyšek to speak the lines for me so I could mark the inflections on the script and know how to say them.

When Čermaková speaks to the headmaster, she gets a few words wrong and he corrects her. And throughout the caning, whenever she lapses into English, he insists she speak Czech. Being forced to adopt the language of my oppressor is powerfully erotic for me. I'd said so in one of my forum posts, unaware that Pavel was taking notes.

At last it was time for my long-awaited caning. The girls fastened the straps, securing me to the bench. People (and legislators) are often disturbed when they see girls tied up for severe punishments, but it's actually much safer. The restraints ensure you can't escape, but they also ensure you won't leap out of position and get hit somewhere damaging. You can't put your hands back or kick your feet in the way. I've had my toes inadvertently hit before; I don't recommend it.

People also fail to realise that we can yell 'Cut!' at any time. Of course, if that did happen, the producer would try to encourage the girl to stay and go through with it (especially if costly footage had already been shot with her), but no one would risk criminal charges by forcing her. However sadistic it may look on film, no one I've worked for is into true non-consensual abuse of unwilling victims. It's a hot fantasy, but it just doesn't happen in the world of CP films. Informed consent is the order of the day. This is a professional industry like any other, with a lot to lose through such irresponsibility.

It's also true that BDSM play requires a high degree of trust. It's a dangerous game and any implement can cause damage if used incorrectly. There's a special thrill in risk-taking but, when you know you're in the hands of a master, there's no real fear that you'll be injured. Marked and bruised, yes, but permanently damaged? No. So I put myself in Pavel's hands, knowing I was completely safe.

It was the hardest caning of my life. And at the time of writing, three years on, that hasn't changed. However, every single one of those fifty strokes was confined to the 'sweet spot' – the fleshy part of the cheeks and the undercurve where the bottom meets the thighs. Through it all I was crying out and pleading in both languages. By the end it was the most natural thing in the world to say, 'Ne, prosím!' and other similar entreaties in Czech. But the restraints did their job; not a single stroke went awry. Pavel was so accurate that I was wearing short-shorts on the streets of Prague the next day.

Oddly enough, it was too intense to give me quite the same high I'd felt on the first shoot. I don't even remember the breaks in between strokes. The pain was overwhelming and I wilted with relief when it was over. But I still had the haircut to come. By then I was eager to be rid of the big hair. Magda had used a ton of mousse and hairspray to hold the style in place and it was looking pretty dishevelled by the end of the caning. It was high summer and I was pouring with sweat. We all were. I was naked, but Pavel was wearing a tailcoat and the other girls were in formal period dresses with pantaloons and heavy stockings.

The crew spent a long time setting up for the haircut because we had only one chance to get it right. I had recovered a bit by this time. The immediacy of the pain was fading and the warm afterglow was starting to set in. Pavel asked how I was. I felt a little dazed, but I was focused enough to express my one worry about the haircut scene. I told him to pull my hair very hard so there could be no doubt that it wasn't a wig. *Make it look real*, I heard my childhood self whispering across the years.

'Like this?' he asked, giving me a savage yank that made my eyes water.

'Uh-huh,' I choked out.

A forced haircut is not something you can do often and not something you can fake if you want the authentic experience. And, prepared as I was, it was still a harrowing ordeal, and one of the most intense roleplays I've ever done. In a way I think it was actually more painful than the caning.

No one had thought to sharpen the blades of the antique scissors, so Pavel couldn't just snip away like a barber. He grabbed a shock of hair, wrenching my head up roughly while the girls held me in place. I felt the rusty scissors struggling to cut through and finally the hair drifted down in front of me. It felt like he was tearing it out rather than cutting it.

And yet . . . I was so aroused. Helpless and ashamed, I was the focus of everyone's attention. At that point in the story you're not meant to feel sorry for me. I'm getting exactly what I deserve for leading these innocent girls astray. It was almost unbearably erotic. At first I struggled and protested, but once my hair was ruined there was no point in fighting any more. I surrendered and wept pitifully while the headmaster completed Čermaková's humiliation. I felt like a World War II collaborator, stripped, beaten and shorn by angry villagers eager to brand me as a sexual traitor. Oh, but that humiliation was *exquisite*.

I think the crew were a bit shocked by the scene. They had to be wondering how on earth Thomas and Pavel had found a girl to do it. But they had fun filming some close-up, slow-motion shots of locks of hair falling to the floor.

It's a fascinating and artistic scene in the final cut. Čermaková crouches naked on the floor, crying, while the lights around her slowly begin to dim. She looks down at the hair in horrified disbelief while a pumping heartbeat swells on the soundtrack and four pairs of shoes slowly back away from her into the shadows. She succumbs to her tears and sinks to the floor, whimpering. It's a scene I'm very proud of.

When it was over, Cameron gathered up all the hair and saved it. 'We can sell it on eBay.'

My bottom was sore, my scalp was tingling, I was sticky with sweat and covered in itchy hair. I had never wanted a shower so desperately in my life. And I couldn't help wondering what I was going to tell the hairdresser when I got home and went to get my hair fixed.

And wouldn't you know it? I still get emails asking whether it was a wig.

(journal entry, age 23)

I thought I saw my dad today. In the club.

I was on stage dancing to something the DJ picked – 'Good Girls Don't, But I Do'. I was on my knees under the strobe light, peeling off my top. I looked up and there he was. Watching me.

I froze.

His stare crucified me. Daddy's little girl was writhing half-naked on a stage with men pawing at her and shoving dollar bills inside her thong. I was everything that disgusted him. I felt the shame like a knife, gutting me.

How could he ever meet my eyes again without seeing me like that? Like all those women in movies he found distasteful, changing the channel with a noise of disapproval. The ones he subliminally begged me not to be.

Then he stepped forwards and smiled and I heaved a sigh of relief. It wasn't him. Just some guy in a nondescript suit and tie who didn't remotely look like my father.

It's not the first time this has happened and I'm sure it won't be the last. He's always there.

But I can't be his little girl and me at the same time. One of us has to go.

9. HOOKER WITH A HEART OF DARKNESS

'I 've never told anybody this before . . .'
    My ears prick up.

'But I . . . well . . .' He trails off, embarrassed. I can tell he's
made this confession before and been rejected. Or ridiculed.

'Yes?'

He chases the last drop of whisky from his glass and sets it on
the table decisively. 'I like feet.'

I blink. Feet. Not choirboys or German shepherds or asphyxi-
ation. Feet.

He misreads my surprise and looks away in frustration. 'Sorry,'
he murmurs.

'Oh no,' I say hurriedly. 'It's just not what I was expecting.
What's so weird about a foot fetish?' I had been hoping he'd say
he wanted to put me over his knee.

With a shrug he turns back to me and his eyes flick down to my
legs. 'Every girl I've ever told has thought it was sick.'

I can't help but laugh. 'They should hear what *I'm* into!'

He relaxes into a grin. 'What is that?'

Now it's my turn to blush as I share my kink with him.

'But . . . I thought you were a dominant,' he says.

My eyes widen. 'Me? But you've seen me dance on stage in a
school uniform!'

'I really only notice the feet,' he admits, as though it's a crime.

I never forgot that conversation. And I heard a lot of confessions in the dark club. They say whores and bartenders make the best therapists. I guess strippers are somewhere in between.

Though I'd always wanted to be an actor, my Hollywood dreams were thwarted by a crippling fear of living among strangers. It was why I'd stayed at home instead of going away to college. I wanted to escape my parents; I just didn't have the courage to run that far. It's one of my biggest regrets.

I was 23 when I finally decided I had to be on my own. The incident with Jessie and Steve had given me the push I needed and I was desperate to find out who I was and where I belonged. I knew what I was into, but I wouldn't discover the Net and the spanking community itself for another year.

On a reckless impulse, I moved into an apartment with three guys I knew casually. It was in the kind of neighbourhood where screams and gunshots are nothing unusual. My parents were horrified. I got a full-time job as an office temp and a part-time job at a video store, so I was rarely even there.

One night I came home to a crime scene. The parking lot was full of cop cars, their red and blue lights splashed across the complex. For once I was spared the death metal that usually blasted from a neighbour's window as I made my way around the building, fearing the worst. The apartment opposite ours had yellow tape across the open front door. POLICE LINE: DO NOT CROSS. One of my roommates told me I'd missed all the excitement. Domestic disturbance. Gunfire.

Another time I got up to find one of my roommates chopping lines on the coffee table. I'd never done coke, but I knew enough to be alarmed by the amount. It was a testament to my naivety that I hadn't known he was a dealer. I had to get out of there. I needed escape money and I needed it fast.

I was proving a miserable failure at office work. (I had problems with authority. Imagine that.) So I decided to follow my exhibitionistic heart and find a job where I didn't have to hide who I was. Flaunting myself was something I could do and do well. It was exactly what my low self-esteem needed.

The first time I went on stage I had no idea what to do. I could barely walk in my borrowed stiletto heels, let alone dance. I was trembling with stage fright and I instantly regretted the complicated corset dress I'd worn. Why hadn't I practised taking it off at home first?

I managed to struggle out of the dress eventually, ignoring the titters of the other girls. I completed the disaster by stumbling in my heels and falling to my knees on the stage. Tears stung my eyes and I reassured myself that it couldn't possibly get any worse. Crashing and burning is sometimes part of the ride. So I picked myself up and limped off stage to some perfunctory applause. It was an inauspicious debut, but I made an encouraging amount of money in tips. Mostly out of pity, I suspect.

I was determined not to give in. All I needed was practice and it wasn't long before I could walk as easily in spike heels as I could barefoot.

Being on stage gave me a performance outlet and table dances paid ridiculously well. In one night I made almost $700, enough for a deposit on my own place. Dancing for a room full of lonely horny men made me feel sexy and confident. I was the centre of attention, grinding against the brass pole and displaying my body under the lights. Men crept to the edge of the stage like supplicants, offering me dollar bills while I towered above them in my five-inch heels. I was their whole world. Every insecure college girl should experience the thrill of being a sex goddess.

I loved dancing. But to my surprise what I loved most was being a trusted confidante. 'Tell me your deepest secret fantasy' was my ice-breaker. I never really expected men to be that open with me. But I was genuinely interested and plenty of them were happy to have someone they could confide in. 'She likes the weirdos,' I overheard another dancer say about me once. I simply preferred the company of fellow misfits.

The foot fetishist paid me to let him massage my feet and suck my toes. My feet are an erogenous zone, so he was almost too good to be true. I couldn't understand why his wife thought it was disgusting, but at least she tolerated his dalliances with dancers. They had a deal; as long as there was no sex it was OK. He felt better not having to sneak around.

I imagined my own version – a boyfriend who wasn't into spanking, but who tolerated the marks other men left on my bottom. No. That would never be enough for me. Nor would I ever be happy with a guy who was willing to do it, but who wasn't into it. That I knew from experience. I'd had guys play along before and it always left me feeling pathetic and unsatisfied. The kinky equivalent of a pity fuck.

Oddly enough, though I often acted the naughty schoolgirl on stage, I seemed to attract submissive men. Occasionally *very* submissive men. I suspect they sensed the kink in me, just not which side of it I was on.

Ted was my first. He tipped me on the main stage, where I was dancing to 'Don't Fear the Reaper'. He said I seemed dark and mysterious and he asked me to join him at his table.

'May I call you "Mistress"?' he asked.

'Uh . . . sure,' I said uncertainly. In my blue velvet hot pants I hardly felt like Mistress material. 'Do you want a dance?'

'Yeah.'

His eyes had a glazed look and he didn't seem all that interested in the usual stripper repertoire. I unveiled my breasts as I slid my hips back and forth in undulating figure eights, but he only watched my face. OK, so he wasn't a breast man. I turned around and slid the hot pants down, exposing my bottom, but he still wasn't really watching. No ass man either. His heavily lined face was set in an expression of either submissive adoration or misery and he made unblinking eye contact any time I was facing him. Unnerved, I had to pretend he was blind just to get through the dance.

He waited until it was over and he'd paid me my twenty dollars to tell me what he really wanted.

'Put your spike heel in my crotch, Mistress,' he whispered.

'What?'

'Please. I'll pay you double.'

I gently rested my foot on his lap, thinking perhaps he was another foot man.

'Press down. Hard.'

I applied a little pressure with the ball of my foot, but Ted shook his head in frustration.

'Your heel,' he gasped. 'Please, Mistress!'

I don't know how or why I complied. It wasn't the money. I suppose I trusted that it was what he wanted and therefore it shouldn't bother me. He shuddered with pain and ecstasy and begged me to slap him across the face.

Again I complied, but it wasn't hard enough for him. So I did it again. This time I hit him as hard as I could.

'More! Harder!'

I glanced nervously around the room. We were alone, so I did it. I slapped him several times in rapid succession, making my hand sting. Then I jammed my stiletto into his crotch again.

'Ohh, yes, Mistress,' he moaned, writhing under my deadly shoe.

Ted became a regular customer. His needs were simple enough, but I was uncomfortable with the whole thing. Afterwards he would slink into the gents to masturbate and then slink back out to humiliate himself further by telling me how inadequate he was.

It made me feel tainted. I didn't like being abusive and nasty. But how could I be so judgemental? Surely it was no different from my desire to be spanked. It was his fantasy, as deeply ingrained in him as my own was in me. Eventually he found another dancer who had no problem being truly sadistic with him. I was relieved.

The oddest request I ever got was from a man who said he liked golden showers. I had no idea what that was, but it sounded interesting.

'It's when you piss on someone,' my customer said cheerfully. 'Or someone pisses on you.'

'Oh.'

Obviously we couldn't do that in the club. He didn't seem to notice my greenish cast as I listened to what he suggested as an alternative. He wanted me to take his empty wineglass into the restroom and fill it up. So he could drink it.

'Gosh, that's not really my thing,' I stammered at last, trying to let him down gently. I was hyper-aware of how painful rejection could be, having experienced it enough myself. He was a sweet guy and I couldn't stand the idea of making him feel like a freak.

Fortunately, he laughed. 'Don't feel bad,' he said. 'It grosses most girls out.'

I did get a spanking one day. Brian was an airline pilot who told me all about his fantasy of a threesome with his wife and a male flight attendant. I liked his honesty and adventurous spirit, so I told him about wanting to be spanked. He seemed excited by the prospect, which in turn excited me. We went to a table in the back room, where he pulled me across his lap and gave me a few gentle love taps. All very mild and playful.

Embarrassed, I giggled and squirmed over his lap, feeling the bulge in his trousers. His arousal turned me on and I made bratty comments to get him to smack me harder. He obliged, laying on a few resounding swats that made me yelp. It hurt, but I didn't feel punished. It wasn't a roleplay and it wasn't authentic, but it was still a welcome drop of water in the desert.

When he threatened to take his belt off I turned scarlet. 'You wouldn't dare,' I said, hoping he would.

Brian smiled. 'I think it's just what a bad girl needs.' He stood up and made a big show of unbuckling the thick leather belt. Then he pulled it through the loops, the loud snicking sound making the blood rush to my head. My face burned as he sat down again, winding the leather around his fist and patting his knee.

I placed myself obediently over his lap again and he gave me several sharp swats with the end of the strap. This was heaven.

He bought four dances from me, squeezing and pinching the reddened skin of my bottom as I straddled him, grinding on his lap and body-sliding down his front. Strippers often tell their customers they're aroused, but this time I didn't have to lie. It was more than obvious to him. The thing that excited me most of all was the simple fact that spanking me had excited *him*. We had to kill some time chatting about the weather before he could get up from the table to say goodbye. I sat there for a while after he'd gone, playing the little scene over and over in my mind.

'I'm surprised you can sit!'

I looked up to see Vanessa, my favourite waitress, grinning at me. She'd heard plenty of confessions herself, including mine.

'You saw that?' I asked, blushing.

'Saw it?' She laughed. 'No, sweetie, but the whole club *heard* it!'

5. Content:

The content (film and stills) we will be shooting will depict scenarios at differing levels and strengths of Spanking and Punishment using the following: Hand, Strap, Paddle and Cane. Punishments will be delivered by fully clothed Male Doms and possibly fully naked Models.

All Models should expect to receive good thrashings. You will return to the USA with marked and bruised buttocks with welts. We think it is important to warn you about this prior to booking so that there is no misunderstanding. Only experienced Spanking Models should take this contract on.

We also require to be able to photograph and film you in explicit positions which will reveal on many occasions your full genitalia.

10. THE GREAT AMERICAN GIRL PROJECT

'Are we ready to start?' asks Dino.

Four schoolgirls look worriedly at the swimming pool. Rosaleen Young was once famously caned holding her ankles at the edge of this pool. More than once, the strokes made her lose her balance and she toppled into the water. All her idea, of course; Rosaleen was her own writer/director. And the video is one of her best. A girl caned in wet schoolgirl knickers – what more could a guy want? But, even though the pool is indoors, the blast of icy air from the open window reminds me that it's January in Yorkshire. I don't really fancy a dip.

'Dino?'

'Yes, Lauren?'

'Are you gonna make us go in the water?'

I can tell by her apprehensive tone she's as unhappy about the prospect as I am. I'm glad someone else asked first.

'If you're up for it,' he replies hopefully.

My eyes widen. 'Um . . .'

He sighs. 'Yes, Niki?'

'I can't swim.'

Darling and Venus look surprised and I hear someone stifle a laugh.

'It *is* bloody cold, Dino,' Shanelle says, coming to my rescue. I'd forgotten that was Shanelle under the nun's habit.

He sighs again and rubs his temples. 'Fine,' he says grudgingly. 'You don't have to go in the pool.'

I begin to relax. A swimming lesson with Sister Mary seemed an implausible premise anyway. Dino and Peppe confer and their alternative seems to suit their personal tastes even more. Sister Mary will strip the four girls and inspect them by the pool *before* their swimming lesson, to make sure they're clean.

Lauren isn't bothered; she's a porn star. And Venus and Darling – well, they've done similar things before. But I feel like I've eaten a spider.

'OK,' I say, not wanting to be difficult. 'But I need to use the loo first.'

Dino's eyes light up. 'Can you do it on camera?'

Everyone's kink is different. Everyone's kink is OK, even if it isn't my kink. I had to remind myself of this many times.

Spanking Online (SOL) is a huge operation with several different websites, spanning several countries. It's run by two brothers – Dino and Peppe – and let's just say their tastes are not confined to spanking.

But they have a reputation for producing some of the best English schoolgirl scenes around. So when David Pierson at spreview.net suggested I be a part of the 'Great American Girl Project', I was tempted. SOL had just done a shoot with several girls in a large country house in Yorkshire and Dino was keen to do it again, this time with American girls.

Venus and Darling were stars of the LA spanking scene. Lauren Legends had done some spanking films, but she was primarily a mainstream porn star and professional escort. David was flying in as well, to cover the event for his website. I couldn't say no.

The contract didn't discuss specific scenarios or storylines, so I had no idea what to expect. My limits tend to be psychological ones rather than physical ones and I was very clear in email about what I would and would not do.

Two of my hard limits are the 'caught smoking' and 'caught masturbating' offences. The first: intense personal aversion. The second: well, it's just nobody else's business what you do alone in your bed and the idea of being punished for it offends me. I've never understood how anyone could realistically *get* caught, anyway. I also told them I'd prefer not to do any scenes where I had to pretend I was enjoying it. 'I'm not that good an actress,' I explained. 'I don't think I could fake that!'

It was a short list, but I still worried that I was being demanding. I was 'the Lupus girl', which gave me a kind of rarified mystique in the industry. But I didn't want anyone to think I was a prima donna. By the end of the shoot, that list would be a lot longer.

The size of the house meant that they could do more than one scene at a time. There was no script; it would all be roleplay and improv. The crew consisted of a single cameraman, sound man and director on each little shoot. It was a much more casual and laidback atmosphere than I was used to at Lupus. But, as I would later learn, that was the norm.

Most of the clips were fairly routine punishment scenarios: headmistress and schoolgirl; aunt and niece; husband and wife. Dino had told us to bring lots of different outfits, as we'd be shooting a variety of scenarios. In addition, he had asked for our measurements so they could provide matching school uniforms. In spite of the careful planning, the measurements got lost and the uniforms they provided were enormous on us. The white cotton school knickers were like diapers and I made a note to myself to provide my own underwear on any future shoots.

Shanelle was the female top hired for the project. A leggy Yorkshire redhead, she was delightfully easy to play off, as she had a response to every bratty comeback. My first scene was with Lauren. We were American students sent to school in England and Shanelle was our headmistress. We had fun playing with the 'American girl' dynamic, rebelling against the uniform and insisting that we didn't know how to knot our ties.

Lauren tossed her blond hair haughtily. My own hair was boyishly short; it hadn't yet recovered from the *Crime and Punishment* shoot. I'd also bleached it in a misguided attempt not to look like the notorious spanking model Niki Flynn.

Lauren rolled her eyes. 'No one wears uniforms in America.'

'You're not *in* America, you silly girl,' Shanelle retorted. 'And I've had enough of your cheek.'

That made me snigger.

'Is something funny, young lady?'

'No,' I said.

'No *what*?'

'No, miss,' I said, rolling my eyes at Lauren.

'Man, all this "sir" and "miss" stuff,' Lauren muttered. 'It's like some big power trip.'

'Keep digging, young lady,' Shanelle said, crossing her arms and smiling coldly. 'You're about to find out what a dose of the cane feels like across your insolent American bottom.'

And she did. Poor Lauren. I don't think she'd ever been caned before. She was pretty shell-shocked and I was glad Cameron was there to comfort her while I took my stripes.

The Brits had all made such a big deal about the American girls having to face the dreaded English cane. But it was only Lauren who was facing something unfamiliar. Darling and Venus and I were genuine enthusiasts, so we were well acquainted with all the implements. It's a shallow assumption in the spanking scene that American girls prefer the paddle and English girls prefer the cane. Personally, I find the American school scene lacking. The formality and ritual of the English one is so much more evocative.

Lauren has a gorgeous bottom, absolutely made for smacking. Shanelle administered a very light caning by industry standards. And Lauren did her best, but it was clear she was struggling. Afterwards she offered Dino a deal: she'd do more sexual things in exchange for less punishment. I was fine with that; it meant I could put my foot down on things *I* didn't want to do.

And I did.

The pool scene with Sister Mary was not my idea of a hot fantasy. Especially as Dino began to embellish the plot with increasing perversion. Each girl would have to bare her bottom for Sister Mary. During the inspection, she would decide that one girl hadn't properly attended to her personal hygiene and so she'd instruct another girl to remedy it. With her tongue. Fortunately, Venus and Darling volunteered.

After the anal tongue bath we had to bend over, one by one, for a strapping. Dino directed the cameraman to lie on the floor behind us, to shoot close-ups. There was even a special light they put behind us so nothing was left to the imagination. I bore all this with gritted teeth, but I pushed back when Dino wanted us to hold our cheeks apart – *wide* apart.

I was beginning to feel like a real prude. But I had thought I was here to shoot spanking scenes, not – well, oral sex and toilet videos. (It became a running joke that whenever anyone went to the loo we'd all yell, 'Cameraman!')

After the pool scene Peppe asked David if he would do a scene with Shanelle and me. I was happy with that. David is a true spanko. So is Shanelle. A scene with the three of us was bound to be much more to my taste.

David played my distraught guardian, a kindly man who seeks the advice of Shanelle because he just doesn't know how to handle his rebellious—

'No, you can't say "daughter"!' Peppe said, stopping the camera.

David and I blinked at each other in surprise. 'What?'

'No mention of mothers or fathers or daughters.'

'We did an aunt/niece scene earlier,' I said.

'That's different.'

Baffled, we let it go.

'What am I supposed to call her, then?' David asked.

'Just call her "my Niki",' he said.

Somehow that sounded even more suggestive.

'I just don't know what to do,' David said, wringing his hands. 'My Niki is out of control. She won't listen to me.'

'Well, I think I can help you, Mr Pierson,' Shanelle said, looking me up and down. 'What girls need is old-fashioned discipline.'

'You mean . . . (gasp) spanking?'

It was a cheesy little scene, but it was a lot of fun to do. And I was happy to play with David. He spanked me with deliberate incompetence and Shanelle took over, demonstrating the proper way to get through to a girl like me. A hard spanking and caning later, I was contrite and sniffling. David gave me a hug and I promised him I would be a good girl. He was so convincing as the well-meaning guardian that I actually got choked up. He held me tightly until Peppe yelled, 'Cut!' To break the serious mood, I bit David's neck.

Peppe froze, looking at us strangely. 'That was really sick,' he said.

Go figure.

11. GIRLS KICK ASS

Rosaleen Young needed no introduction. Not to a spanko, anyway. The diminutive star had her own website and legions of fans.

I had actually met her once before, at a party in London. We chatted for a while and then she apparently overheard me telling Cameron that I was dying to cane someone. I'm not really a switch, but I do enjoy using the cane. Unfortunately, Rosaleen didn't have the courage to volunteer that night.

She came to the house to shoot some material for her website. This time she had all the courage and I had none.

'You want me to top you?' I gulped. 'On camera?'

'You'll be brilliant!'

I was very insecure, but I'm not one to turn down a new experience. 'Well,' I said. 'I can't really take myself seriously as an authority figure.'

'How about playing a bully, then?'

I thought about it. I had roleplayed an abusive prefect before, who then got her own comeuppance for caning another girl without permission. Cameron and I had done that scene with friends. It was the best of both worlds – getting to use the cane on someone and then having it used on *me*.

'Sure, I think that will work.'

She suggested we be sisters. That sounded good, though I worried about the implication that we had parents, given SOL's special paranoia. She scoffed at that and said she never worried about it.

And so, wearing my 'Girls kick ass' T-shirt, I played the bullying older sister. Rosaleen wore her long dark hair in two plaits, instantly taking years off her real age. I was self-conscious enough about my unfortunate yellow hair; next to Rosaleen I felt like the ugly stepsister!

'Ex*cuse* me,' the imperious little madam said as she marched into the room in her stripey red bra and white hot pants. 'This is *my* room!'

'It's my room now,' I sneered, tossing her mobile phone onto the floor.

'Hey! That's my phone! What were you doing, trying to steal my boyfriend's messages?'

'Yeah, I wanted to see all the dirty numbers you call.'

'How dare you!'

She launched herself at me on the bed and we struggled until I wrestled her across my knee. 'Whose room is it now?' I demanded.

'It's *my* room!'

She wouldn't give in. So I brought my hand down on her bottom. Hard. I alternated from the left cheek to the right, until my palm began to sting. Rosaleen yelped at every smack, pretending my delicate little hand was hurting her. She egged me on, calling me names to make me hit her harder. I did my best, but it was agony.

When my hand just couldn't take any more I ran my nails over her pinkened cheeks, tickling her and making her squeal and thrash around. I switched to my left hand when my right one stung too much, teasing her with my nails when I needed a break. This was so much more work than being the spankee!

The hot pants were adorable and I hated to take them down, but I knew the viewers would be disappointed not to see her bare cheeks. I began another onslaught, still hurting my hands more than her rock-hard bottom, and then stopped to ask her again whose room it was.

'My room,' she said through gritted teeth.

It was a perfect scene for an uncertain top. Rosaleen could just keep insisting it was her room until she'd had enough. I'd stop when she gave in. No need for any clumsy safewords. I felt a little more secure and let her have it, laying on with a will while she kicked and protested.

Finally, I twisted her arm up behind her back and gave her a last volley of extremely hard swats, trying not to wince with pain myself.

'It's so unfair,' she moaned.

'Yes it is,' I said brightly. 'But whose room is it?'

She pouted for a moment before muttering, '*My* room.'

My poor hands had to endure more abuse before she finally surrendered.

'OK, OK, it's your stupid room!'

'Good,' I said, letting her up. 'Then get your stuff out of it.'

She ran off in a huff and I looked at my palms. They were bright red with purple bruises. Venus topped her later in another scene and remarked, 'Dude, I spanked that girl's butt so hard I bruised my hand!' I could definitely sympathise.

Rosaleen is the consummate professional, both on and off camera. During our scene she moved seamlessly between her actress and director roles, stopping mid-yelp to give directions to the cameraman and slipping right back into character.

After the scene was over she asked if I'd do another one with her.

'Oh no!' I wailed. 'My hands can't take any more!'

She laughed. 'No, I mean, let's do one where we get spanked together.'

That sounded fun to me, so I suggested a pillow fight. Rosaleen loved it and told the cameraman to start rolling. We had a blast hitting each other with pillows and shrieking with laughter. A large wardrobe stood beside the bed and at one point she shoved me against it very hard. I was afraid it was going to fall on us. The noise woke our housemistress.

'I'm not surprised you didn't hear me,' Shanelle said when we finally noticed her looming over us, 'with the noise you two are making.'

Niki: (innocently) We were just going to bed, miss.

Rosaleen: Yeah, just saying our prayers.

Shanelle: I've heard nothing but noise, giggling and banging.

Niki: I fell out of bed.

Rosaleen: She did, miss. I was just helping her back in.

Shanelle: (sarcastically) I see, so I walked in just as you were picking her up off the floor. With a pillow.

Niki: The pillows fell too.

Shanelle: The pillows fell too. One in each hand?

Rosaleen: (chirpily) We wanted to make the bed nice and neat before we went to sleep.

Shanelle: It seemed that way to me as well when I walked in and two pillows were right up in the air, just about to land on each other's heads.

We collapsed into giggles at that point. For some reason, the housemistress didn't buy our story. One at a time she put us across her knee for a hard spanking. When both our bottoms were red and sore, Shanelle finished with another scolding, asking us if we were sorry, if we'd learned our lesson and were ready to go to bed now – without falling out.

We promised we would. Then Rosaleen said, 'Fuck you very much, miss,' when she was meant to thank Shanelle for the spanking. I managed not to crack up, but only just barely. Shanelle apparently didn't notice. She said good night; we crawled into bed and, as soon as she was out of sight, the pillows flew again.

The scene ended with each of us over a knee, our bottoms almost touching while Shanelle used both hands to spank us. Definitely a crowd-pleaser.

When it was all over I noticed a long red scratch down the length of my right arm where I had scraped it on the wardrobe.

Rosaleen was dismayed. 'It's bleeding!'

It was pretty funny, really. After two days of being thrashed non-stop, the only thing I had to show for it was a scratch I gave myself. I still have the scar.

12. CONFESSION

The grand finale of the Great American Girl Project convinced David that we were all going to hell. Both he and Venus had gone to Catholic school, so the profane story Dino proposed had them exchanging nervous sidelong glances. It sounded innocent enough at first. Sister Mary was to hear confessions from us and then give us penance – with her strap and cane. But, predictably, Dino's ideas of confessions were rather smutty.

Darling was first, confiding to Sister Mary that she had impure thoughts. Actually, what Dino wanted her to say was, 'My anus seeps juices.' Someone murmured that Dino had a lot to learn about female anatomy.

'Impure thoughts? Ah, that's a grave sin, my child,' said Shanelle, lapsing into an Irish accent.

'Cut! You can't say "child" in a video,' Dino instructed.

Shanelle gawped at him. 'How the bloody hell can I be a nun and not say "my child"?'

'Just try,' Dino pleaded. 'Right. "Catholic Anus", take two.'

Venus and David shuddered.

Darling's penance was a severe strapping. Shanelle had her kneel on the floor with her bottom raised up high so that everything was on display. Then she took off the crucifix she was wearing and handed it to Darling. 'Hold this and pray to the Lord for forgiveness, my child.'

Dino flinched and I had to bite my tongue to keep from laughing.

The strapping was long and hard and Darling prayed fervently the whole time, looking earnestly heavenwards. And, afterwards, Dino asked her if she could masturbate while saying the Lord's Prayer. As one does.

'I don't understand the logic,' Cameron whispered to me. 'You can't say "parents" or "my child", but blasphemy is fair game?'

It was a stunning performance. And, while I never saw the finished video, I'd love to see Darling's prayer again. Her moans and gasps were remarkably authentic and the whole thing was so obscene I half expected us all to be struck by lightning. It was like watching a train wreck. An inexplicably erotic one.

Venus shook her head in amazement and took Darling's place. She confessed to lusting after the other girls in the changing room. Her penance was a caning and Sister Mary instructed her to say a Hail Mary after each cane stroke. The words flowed over her tongue with practised ease and when it was over she laughed and said, 'Damn! I haven't prayed that hard since Catholic school!'

Finally, it was my turn. Dino wanted me to confess to self-abuse. One of my hard limits.

'You don't actually have to *do* it,' he assured me. 'Just confess to it.'

I didn't want to give ground, but I couldn't think of an alternative. And I wasn't about to let Dino suggest something else. We all have undiscovered limits and Dino seemed to have a knack for finding mine. So I relented. Whatever I confessed to was going to be anticlimactic after Darling anyway. However, my meek 'Sometimes I touch myself' wasn't rude enough for Dino. He insisted I use the word 'vagina'.

'Dino, no girl would ever say that!' I laughed. 'Trust me.'

Darling and Venus echoed agreement, but there was no dissuading him. He's very particular about his kinks. Fair enough; so am I.

So I made my vulgar confession and took my punishment. Sister Mary instructed me to pray for forgiveness and I froze. Me? Pray? What was I supposed to say? I had claimed in my interview with David that I was raised Catholic, but I couldn't pull it off here. I muddled through a lame and unconvincing plea for mercy and was relieved when it was over. I just had to hope no one would notice.

* * *

It was done. Almost. SOL wanted to do one more little scene. Dino gave each of us eight strokes of the cane before calling in Elizabeth Simpson. Elizabeth had been a spanking video star for years, but had taken some time off. She hadn't been topped in over a year.

Now she was ready to dive in again and she wanted to show the Yanks what English girls were made of. Bending over the bed, she took a strapping that made our eyes water. Then it was time for the cane. It was one of the heaviest canings I'd seen, but she didn't make a sound. In fact, she was so stoic that Peppe, who was filming, prompted her for some reaction.

'Oww,' she said sarcastically.

When it was over she straightened herself up, readjusted her uniform and beamed at all of us. 'Simpson is back!' she declared.

Dino turned to his American guests. 'One last offer,' he said. 'I'll give any of you an extra $20 per stroke if she'll take a caning like that.'

'No fuckin' way!' Venus said, crossing her arms.

Darling shook her head. 'Sorry, Dino. Not me.' She was so severely bruised that another caning might draw blood.

But I couldn't resist. It wasn't the money and it wasn't just the opportunity to show off, though I did want my chance after seeing Elizabeth's display. No, it was that silly English myth that American girls don't like the cane. And Dino's insinuation that we couldn't take it.

I adopted the same position Elizabeth had, bending over the bed. David loves to tell the story of how Dino gave in before I did. It was hard, but it was only four strokes.

Afterwards, I got shakily to my feet and rubbed my sore bottom.

'So,' Dino said, grinning smugly. 'Would you like to move to England?'

I didn't hesitate. 'Yeah!'

Guten Tag, Niki!

Your films have always been for me a big inspiration. I love to see you acting.

I always get very sexually aroused when I spank a woman. I think most of the spanking sessions in real life are ending with sex.

I have a big question. Perhaps you can answer this question to me, because you are an "insider". Why do not spanking films end with hot sex, which both actors enjoy? I think that such a film produced by Rigid East/Lupus would be a bestseller.

Liebe Grüße,

Kurt, Berlin

13. LET'S TALK ABOUT SEX

O K, I promised. Sex.
A lot of people like their spankings to lead to sex. And
erotic spankings with a slow build-up and lots of fondling can be
very nice. There are a few film companies who make consensual
sex part of the story. I have nothing against mutually pleasurable
stimulation that gets both partners hot and bothered. But ultimately it's not my kink. It doesn't fit my punishment/abuse
fantasies and it's inauthentic in a disciplinary setting.

Non-consensual sex is another matter. And the more daring
companies don't shy away from that particular fantasy. The sex
itself is faked and it's more a dramatic plot element than a
prurient 'money shot'. As a girl who grew up on rape and snuff
fantasies, I applaud filmmakers who are brave enough to embrace
such scenes.

My first real sexual experience was with a girl. Her name was
Julia. She was a stripper and she was always trying to convince
me to go with her to the club. But, at that point in time, stripping
was something I couldn't even imagine doing. I had just turned 21
and I still lived with my parents. I was far too insecure. And
terrified of what my parents would think if they found out. My
mother had been shocked enough to learn that I'd applied for a
waitress job at Hooters, where the girls wear tight white cotton
crop-tops and orange hot pants. (They didn't hire me; I had no
waitressing experience.)

One night Julia was showing me some moves at my boyfriend's apartment. The same boyfriend I had tried to share *Frank and I* with. Roger's most adventurous fantasy was 'two chicks', so this kind of show was a dream come true for him.

I was still a virgin. I had messed around, but I had this archaic notion of saving myself for marriage. Julia and I were a little drunk and Roger was cheering us on. So, before we knew it, we were giving him the kind of show he'd always fantasised about. Julia was the aggressor and at one point she twisted her hand in my hair, pulled my head back and bit my neck. *That* was exciting for me. But, though I kept presenting my bottom to her, she didn't pick up the hint. Instead of smacking me, she merely caressed me and slipped her hands in between my legs.

Eventually we lost all our inhibitions and, before I knew it, I was going down on her. Julia had a fast noisy orgasm and then it was my turn. I faked mine. Actually, I've always wondered whether she did too. It was fun, but ultimately I didn't see what all the fuss was about. I'd much rather have been spanked.

A few months later I was single again and I gave my virginity to the first creep who convinced me he was into spanking. In reality, he was into anything that would get a girl into bed with him. I felt duped and betrayed. Most of all I hated myself for having been so gullible.

He called me frigid and said I was afraid of intimacy. Intimacy? That was rich.

I suppose bad sex with bad people would turn anyone off, but for me the separation was more drastic. As I grew older and more experienced I decided that I could happily do without it. I was the perfect stripper because it was so completely impersonal. But, after nearly two years of dancing full-time, I became disillusioned with the club scene. I was tired of being a sex object when I felt just like the opposite. I enjoyed the dance, the tease, but that was it. All I needed was someone who wanted to spank me as much as I wanted to be spanked. And who wouldn't want sex in return.

Sex just made no sense in my fantasies. The headmaster doesn't get all worked up and throw his pupil down on the desk and screw her silly. Daddy's naughty little girl doesn't get horny after he's taken her over his knee for a dose of the hairbrush. I needed to know that my punisher was interested in *punishment*, not foreplay.

And yet it was confusing because I did have sexual responses to spanking fantasies. I did masturbate. Quite a lot. But I never thought about sex when I did; I only thought about spanking.

I suppose I could blame my father. It's a peculiar feature of modern society that parents are often indifferent to televised violence, while prohibiting sex with puritanical zeal. That was certainly true in my case. As a child I was allowed to watch any gruesome horror film I wanted to, but, if people started having sex, my dad would turn it off. He wasn't quick enough with *A Clockwork Orange*, though, and I saw most of the scene where the rival gang strips and paws the 'weepy young devotchka' before he changed the channel.

It was at the height of my disillusionment that I met Cameron. I was in a crumbling relationship with an older man who wasn't the pure spanko he'd led me to believe. Nor was he as non-possessive as he'd claimed. Even with vanilla boyfriends, I was always adamant about one thing: jealousy was a deal-breaker. I'd had my fill of possessive men. Especially the ones who insisted they weren't jealous, had their fun with other girls and then gave me the cold silent treatment when I played with spanko friends. No, I wanted an open relationship with someone I could trust not to treat me like property. Sex was constantly getting in the way. We were becoming increasingly incompatible and I was becoming increasingly bitter and cynical.

Cameron was English, with a public-school accent and natural authority. We found each other through a spanking site online, so there were no awkward confessions about what we were into. He'd asked me for a critique of a spanking story he'd written and my efforts fell short of his expectations. I wasn't critical enough. His response, in schoolmaster mode, was better than any of the CP videos I'd seen. His kink was exactly the same as mine: CP was arousing, but it didn't have to lead to sex. Best of all, he told me he couldn't get aroused at all without the spanking element. Just like me.

We spent a week together, just the two of us. It changed our lives forever.

He fitted me with an authentic school uniform he'd brought from the UK and I felt like a little girl as he taught me how to knot the tie. The ideal English headmaster, he was my fantasy made flesh. He scolded me about my misbehaviour before instructing me to lift my skirt and position myself across a chair. I obeyed, my hands trembling with dread and excitement.

I jumped when I felt his fingers on my white cotton knickers. He didn't pull them down. Instead, he adjusted them carefully, smoothing them across the curves of my bottom. This thorough attention to detail was more embarrassing than taking them off would have been. I felt a little surge of heat between my legs and I squirmed.

At last he laid the cane across the taut school knickers. 'You will count each stroke,' he said. 'Say "Thank you, sir," after each one.'

I held my breath, waiting.

The first stroke made me yelp and I grabbed the edge of the chair for support. I'd been caned before, but never with such precision, such formality. And never by an Englishman. The knickers offered no protection at all and I marvelled at the escalating sting. Whoever devised caning as a punishment definitely knew what they were doing. There's just nothing like it.

'One, thank you, sir.'

He gave me twelve strokes in that scene – six over my knickers and six on the bare. Plus an extra one for miscounting.

Cameron held me afterwards while we talked about the intensity of the scene and shared our favourite moments. I loved his soft-spoken authority and couldn't wait to do another roleplay.

We spent the week playing scene after scene, stopping only to eat and sleep. I was a reformatory girl caned for insolence. A vandal sentenced to a judicial birching. A niece spanked over her strict uncle's knee. I was bruised and sore, but insatiable. We only had this one week; we had to get it all in.

There seemed to be no limit to the places we could go in our heads. Best of all, none of it was tainted by the pressure of having to perform or put out afterwards. The psychodrama was enough. Sexual tension simmered just below the surface, but neither of us needed to act on it. I had never felt so open with anyone in my life.

It's a special kind of intimacy, trusting someone to cause you pain, to push your limits, to take you to an extreme physical and emotional place. And yet knowing at the same time that you're perfectly safe, that you will not be harmed. That afterwards you'll be comforted and told how brave you were. Vanilla sex could never take me anywhere like that.

In one scene Cameron was a Victorian gentleman and he sent his maid to fetch the morning paper for him. I gasped when I saw it – a copy of the London *Times* dated Friday, 19 October 1888. On page 5 was an article about the Whitechapel murders, along with the famous 'From Hell' letter sent to Scotland Yard by Jack the Ripper. I'd casually mentioned my Jack the Ripper fascination in an email weeks before and Cameron had paid attention. It's the quirkiest Valentine anyone's ever given me, and the one I treasure most.

On a subsequent visit we decided to push the boundaries. We did a kidnapping roleplay that overshadowed everything we'd done before. It was a recurring story we dipped in and out of over several days. I was a stripper coming home from work along the alley behind his house. Cameron chased me down, caught me and dragged me inside. I fought, but he was stronger. He subdued me, gagged me and tied me up in the cupboard. When he opened it again ten minutes later he smiled and said, 'Good morning. It's playtime.'

This time I wasn't a girl subject to official discipline from a legitimate authority figure. It wasn't 'fair'. I was his pet, his plaything. He'd caught me and would do what he liked with me. I'd be punished too, when I displeased him. But sometimes I would be punished simply because he felt like spanking or whipping me. He'd removed the parameters of institutionalised discipline. It created a very special headspace and a profound vulnerability in me.

This time the play did start to edge into more sexual territory.

He cut away my clothes with a knife. I moaned and whimpered in shame, pleading with him to let me go. So he gagged me again. He took great delight in inspecting his property. Mortified at his attentions, I squeezed my eyes shut tight, blushing furiously. He led me to the bathroom, where he bathed me, smacking me like a child whenever I didn't cooperate. I was dizzy with powerlessness and when his hands strayed between my legs I felt the violation acutely – as desire. My sexual awakening had begun.

I'd shelved my self-destructive rape fantasies. They were about sex and sex was the enemy. But now all I wanted was for him to take me and have his way with me. In between scenes I hinted that it would be OK, but still he didn't do it. My body ached with need. I didn't understand my sudden longing but, even though I could see he was aroused as well, he confined himself to more punitive delights.

After one scene, Cameron held me and told me how proud he was of me. 'I never thought I would find anyone like you. You have the same fantasies I do, from schoolgirl punishments to capture and rape. You surrender completely in a scene, and I can do whatever I want with you. But after a few hugs you're back to your everyday self, without a submissive bone in your body. You're my perfect complement.'

I was glad he'd said it first; I didn't have the guts. And I couldn't escape the reality: I was falling in love.

The visit was over and we parted like parolees being sent back to prison. I cried all the way home. I tried to downplay the connection we'd made, but my partner could see what had happened. He'd lost me. I moved in with Cameron four months later.

One night not long after I arrived, we were in bed watching *The Night Porter*. The controversial cult movie stars Dirk Bogarde as a former Nazi officer and Charlotte Rampling as his prisoner. Thirteen years after the war, the pair meet again by chance in the Vienna hotel where Bogarde works as a night porter. Haunted by the past, they resume their sadomasochistic love affair.

As in the best horror movies, the power of *Night Porter* lies in the things it doesn't show. The ambiguity forces you to fill in the blanks. And I did.

In one flashback scene, Rampling is chained to the bed and Bogarde puts his hands proprietarily on her breasts. Then he slips two fingers into her mouth and moves them gently in and out. There is no dialogue, but the subtle unspoken show of power and the inherent threat had me squirming. I was right back in the kidnap roleplay.

Seeing my reaction, Cameron tied my hands together and attached the rope to the headboard of the four-poster bed. Then he offered me his finger, guiding it into my mouth. I resisted, but he held my head firmly until I complied. He kept me tied up for the rest of the movie, molesting me while I pretended to hate it.

When the movie was over he continued his explorations. He unbuttoned my shirt to expose me, letting his hands roam over my breasts. I whimpered with embarrassment and strained against the rope as he pinched my nipples. His hand crept lower, down inside my panties. I gasped and struggled. He parted my knees roughly and I felt a rush of excitement.

'That's right,' he said softly. 'You know what happens to disobedient girls, don't you?'

I moaned and shook my head as he slid my panties down.

'They're sent to the punishment room. To be whipped. Is that what you want?'

'No.'

'No what?'

'No, sir,' I gasped, overwhelmed by my body's response.

He went on to tell me how I would be used by the officers, one by one, and that, if I didn't please them or show the proper respect, I would be punished. Severely. I closed my eyes, picturing a room full of officers in smart military uniforms, like the iconic scene in the movie where Rampling sings in German. (I performed that song one night for Cameron wearing a pair of his trousers, braces, black opera gloves and a Royal Navy captain's hat.)

I had no choice. I was to be their whore, their slave, their plaything. They would pass me around and do anything they wanted to with me and there was nothing I could do about it. Resistance would only earn me more punishment.

'Some of the officers,' Cameron continued, 'have very special tastes. I know of one who always asks for girls who have broken the rules. He wants the pleasure of administering their discipline himself.'

My head was spinning as he added layer upon layer of exquisite cruelty to the image he was painting. I hadn't been so turned on since seeing my first CP video. Finally, he turned me over and told me to kneel up.

'Of course, the guards are allowed their fun too. If an officer hasn't chosen you that day, you may be given to one of the guards. A treat for him, a punishment for you. And some of them can be very cruel indeed.'

He gave me a couple of sharp smacks, making me jump. My hands were still tied, so I couldn't reach back. I pleaded with him, but he laughed softly.

'Yes, I know how girls like to try and earn our sympathy,' he said, his voice low and menacing. 'But you wouldn't be here if you hadn't been naughty, would you?'

Finally, when I didn't think I could stand it any longer, he took me from behind. He was very rough and I cried out as he thrust inside me. Every nerve in my body tingled with electricity and he continued to spin fantasies as he fucked me fast and hard. I'd been dreaming of this moment for weeks, ever since the kidnapping. I felt alive in a way I never had before, as though he'd freed a hidden part of me. And he hadn't even spanked me!

Afterwards, I lay panting and gasping in his arms, marvelling that it had taken me so long to find the obvious key. Non-consent. I'd reclaimed my adolescent rape fantasies, only now they weren't self-destructive; they were liberating. This time I was choosing the fantasies rather than having them inflicted on me by a brain I thought was deranged.

Now, at least once a week, I wake up to a soft voice in my ear, telling me all the ways in which I will be debauched and violated. And what will happen to me if I don't comply. When you're with someone you trust completely, someone you can share your deepest secret fears with, nothing is taboo.

Dear Niki,

Keep suffering pain for your pleasure . . . and ours!

Maybe tonight, before going to bed, you could torture the soles of your feet a bit . . . how about oiling them and slightly roasting them with the flame of a candle? Can you imagine going to sleep with red, sore, pulsating roasted soles, the dream you would have?

Just don't roast your arches, as the skin there is more delicate.

Regards

DG, South America

14. NOT MY SOCKS!

I get a lot of emails from guys with specific fantasies and requests. It appeals to the whore in me to be allowed into their minds, to have such a privileged glimpse into their kink.

It's a mistake to assume that people who like spanking are all alike. There is a bewildering array of variations on the theme. But if there's one universal truth about any fetish, it's that *details matter*. In some cases the details are *all* that matters. Fetishists know what they like. I certainly do.

The dress code, for example, always generates debate. The hard-core schoolies (that includes me) demand authentic school uniforms – crisp white shirts and properly knotted ties, regulation skirts and white cotton knickers. They won't be satisfied with a 'schoolgirl' in a crop top, tartan miniskirt, thong and high heels. They also prefer authentic disciplinary scenarios, though they're usually willing to overlook the implausibility of over-the-knee spanking in a school setting.

Of course, there are plenty of viewers who don't care about authenticity or costumes or roleplay. They don't care what the girl wears – and a lot of them prefer her naked. Although I've done it a lot, nudity doesn't really appeal to me in CP movies. There are certainly contexts where it's appropriate, but in general I find it much more embarrassing to have just my bottom bared for punishment. Nudity leaves nothing to the imagination.

One interesting request came from a man whose fantasy involves stripped schoolgirls. He was disappointed that, in many such scenes, the girls kept their socks on. A girl wasn't fully and properly shamed by her nudity, he argued, if she was allowed to retain her socks. Now, I've never found exposing my feet to be especially embarrassing, but I promised to pretend it was mortifying if I was ever ordered to remove my socks.

There is a wide range of preferences over the spankee's reactions too. Most people like a certain amount of whimpering, crying and protesting. And real tears are always a favourite. If a girl is too stoic, there's no way to judge what she's feeling. Is it too much? Not enough? Is she freaked out? Angry? Bored? Least popular of all is a very heavy beating with no reaction from the girl. Guys compare it to pounding a slab of meat.

However, one viewer I know prefers stoic girls; too much crying and screaming puts him off. The noise is not always something a girl can control. Spankings hurt. I think it's hot to see a girl *try* to be stoic, but not succeed.

Some people like a long, slow build-up. They want all the backstory. They want to see the girl sneaking out the door, getting caught, being sent to the headmaster, waiting nervously, being scolded and then being punished. The build-up is often the hottest part. There are plenty of people who don't care at all about the story and just fast-forward to the action. I often do the reverse: watch all the build-up and skip the actual punishment. One of the perks of my job is free spanking porn, so perhaps I need the variety more than most.

Even if it's not my kink, it's arousing to be cast in someone else's fantasy. There's the German man who wants to play doctor. The medical fantasies he shares with me are excruciatingly embarrassing, but somehow they turn me on in spite of myself.

Another man wants to be my daddy. He's not interested in sex and he disapproves of my darker movies; all he wants is to treat me like a little girl and buy me ice cream. Then he'll spank me if I'm naughty and put me to bed. I blush when I read his emails, regressing as I imagine being taken care of like that.

Then there's the guy in South America who likes dirty feet. He wants me to walk around barefoot for a whole weekend – outdoors, in the city streets, on the metro – and then tie me up and whip my dirty soles until I'm screaming in pain and begging him to stop. I can't say it's not my kink because I'm always intrigued by foot fetishists, but I have to draw the line at roasting my soles over a flame.

On the technical side, one man discovered my website while on holiday. He spent his time under the palm trees writing the synopsis of a fourteen-part film series with me as a kinky undercover cop who's always willing to get spanked in the line of duty. Each episode ended with me realising I'd been duped in some way – infiltrated a gang the force wasn't pursuing or suffered 'a series of humiliating punishments' to get evidence they already had. The sting-in-the-tail endings were deliciously reminiscent of the Cheri Caffaro 'Ginger' movies from the 1970s. Ginger was the female James Bond who used her body and insatiable sexual appetite to fight crime, always managing to get captured and tied up along the way.

The requests I enjoy most are the ones with meticulous attention to detail. Exact numbers of strokes and implements, imaginative positions, specific items of clothing . . . I share them with Cameron and sometimes they inspire our own roleplays.

I especially love reading the posts on my Yahoo group from members who devise elaborate scenarios and creative new ways to torture me. They want to see me as a female pirate captain, overthrown by her mutinous crew and flogged at the grating. A faithless wife in the Old West, caught by her husband and bullwhipped by her lover at gunpoint. A woman at the mercy of the Spanish Inquisition, examined and tortured. Their imaginations know no bounds.

I even proposed a scenario of my own for them: a girl discovers an online forum where people have been discussing cruel and evil things to do to her, in gory detail. She contacts a special Internet group that deals with such situations. The group arranges for the members to be kidnapped and given the same treatment they prescribed for the poor innocent girl. Naturally, she gets to watch.

One member added his own twist: the girl discovers too late that the Internet group is actually just a front for the online forum, who kidnap her and then enact the 'cruel and evil things' they had been plotting all along. If it wasn't so hot I suppose it might be creepy.

The idea that I am the manifestation of someone's fantasy is intensely erotic. It's objectifying, and yet it's never depersonalising. I'm sharing myself intimately with the viewer. You project; I reflect. I can be the perfect girl who will never disappoint you. The perfect whore. Sexual fantasy is potent stuff. And to be objectified so intimately is a profound psychosexual experience.

Wonderful movies, for my humble opinion. When I first saw the Lupus videos I had some feeling of . . . dignity. Of course – these are very severe films. But the masochistic actresses seemed to be treated with respect. They suffer, they cry – yes, of course. Exactly. That is the story. But the way in which Lupus films are made shows a certain . . . seriousness, and that means dignity for their actresses.

I would like to express my highest respect to them. They are taking pain and suffering for my personal pleasure. My erotic pleasure. They are giving us (sadistic/dominant people) a valuable gift – their devotion, their passion.

Tom, Germany

15. STALIN 2: HOW TO MAKE A SPY

'Take away everything that gives the prisoner strength to resist – food, sleep, dignity. Take away her senses so that she can't see or hear. Restrain her so that she can't move. Why should you do all the work? Let the prisoner's own body become her enemy – it will ache and torture her. There's no hurry. You have got time. Plenty of time . . .'

Naked from the waist down, I balance unsteadily on an overturned bucket in my cell. The straitjacket immobilises my arms and my legs tremble from the effort of keeping my balance. If I fall they will beat me. Again.

The heavy black bag over my head shuts out my sight, held in place by a rope tied securely around my neck. The only sound is my laboured breathing, harsh and rapid. It takes all my self-control to resist the creeping claustrophobia. If I allow it to set in I'll panic.

A bead of sweat runs down my face and I teeter precariously. With a gasp I recover my balance and manage not to fall. A tiny victory, but I am determined. They won't make me confess to something I didn't do.

'You must bring the prisoner to such a state that she will fear for her own sanity, her own life. Put her into a situation that makes her understand clearly that she can't hold out forever. She will break.'

My eyes widen with fear as they release me and try a new tack. They lock me naked against the wall, my wrists and neck in iron shackles. And when the first trickle of cold water drips onto my head, I feel my sanity begin to slip.

Lupus had trouble finding someone to translate the forty-page script into English for me, so they sent me the Czech version. I worked laboriously through my scenes word by word to see what they were going to do to me. And as my fate became clear I had the eerie sense that they had unlocked my mind and extracted my deepest, darkest fantasies.

Stalin 2: How to Make a Spy was the movie I had been waiting for, the one I had first fantasised about being a part of. Caning, torture, interrogation, brainwashing ... I know, it's not everyone's cup of tea.

What could possibly be eroticised about Stalinist Communism? It bears repeating: there is nothing more erotic than power. And there is a special erotic charge in power *abused*. I love being pushed to scary emotional places. Places where those in power can do anything they want to me. Places where I have no control.

The story focuses on the conspiracy-minded secret police in early 1950s Czechoslovakia and the unfortunates denounced as 'class enemies' by the Communist machine. Conspiracy is the Party's *raison d'être*. It's the StB's job to discover the imperialistic spies. And there must *be* spies or the Party wouldn't mention them. Tyranny flourishes in this kind of twisted logic. So do edgy BDSM films.

Pavel Šťastný says he's always had an erotic attraction to totalitarian regimes because they're the ultimate expression of dominance and submission. One group of people is ruling another with absolute power, creating endless opportunities to exploit and abuse. It's unlikely that StB agents were as perverse as the ones depicted in Lupus films. But that's the beauty of fantasy. It bears little resemblance to the brutal reality; that's the whole point.

In *Stalin 2*, Kateřina Tetová reprises her role from *Stalin*, pleading her innocence to no avail. No one is spared. The form teacher, the headmaster and even the ruthless Communist commissar fall victim to the regime. Two of Kateřina's classmates are also implicated.

My character, Nikolaja, is stubborn and defiant. The StB accuse her of being the ringleader of a western imperialistic conspiracy.

Of course this group doesn't exist, but the StB need a conspiracy to justify their existence and their methods. One by one, the girls give in and confess their involvement. Nikolaja holds out the longest, enduring ever more bizarre and brutal tortures until madness sets in. It's the dilemma faced by the victims of witch trials and the Spanish Inquisition: suffer and hope your endurance will prove your innocence. Or confess and be executed. Not your usual formula for a kinky story, but then Lupus films are rarely prosaic.

16. PORN WITH A POLITICAL AGENDA

Stalin 2 is more than just a CP movie. It's not porn. It's not frivolous entertainment. It's political satire of the blackest kind. At dinner one night, Thomas Marco explained to me that Communism is alive and well in the Czech Republic. Despite the fall of Communism in 1989 (the 'Velvet Revolution'), former StB agents remain in positions of power. Thomas said this was the inspiration for the movie. So it's an act of rebellion. An anti-communist manifesto. The older members of the Lupus cast and crew have very personal and unpleasant memories of the regime. This was a reality they lived.

But ultimately it's still a CP film, aimed at those of us who are wired this way. For me it's the perfect blend of horror and erotica. Even the comedic moments take on a sinister tone, highlighting the cruelty and arbitrariness of the system.

In the climax of the film, the StB think Nikolaja is ready to break, so they deliver her to the Soviet counsellor's office, naked, wet and cold, to give her one last chance to sign the confession. All the agents are there, surrounding her. When she refuses, the counsellor sighs and pulls out a gun. He forces her down over the desk and puts the gun to the back of her head. Trembling, Nikolaja waits in terror, but, when he pulls the trigger, there is only an empty CLICK! Broken at last, she collapses on the floor, hysterically promising to say anything they want her to.

Intense.

Unfortunately, the movie was shot out of sequence, as many are. I'd been caned the day before, but I had yet to experience any of the more inventive tortures promised by the script. And just before the mock execution, Nikolaja is supposed to have been chained to the wall with water dripping on her head for several hours, pushing her to the brink of insanity.

'What's my motivation?' I joked, wondering how I was going to dredge up the emotion. I couldn't help but think of Brandon Lee, accidentally shot and killed on the set of *The Crow*. But that wasn't enough to make me feel my character's terror.

Pavel understood exactly what I needed – to simulate the torture Nikolaja endured just before the scene. He suggested that I go stand under some cold water until they were ready for me. Being cold and wet would help me get inside Nikolaja's head. Cameron had a better idea. He said we should make it into a roleplay, that that would be a more authentic experience in preparation for the scene. You know me and authenticity. Pavel agreed. So they stripped me, handcuffed me and sent me away with Cameron.

'Come on, Nikolaja,' he said, dragging me down the hallway and into the bathroom.

He turned on the cold tap in the sink and splashed me with water, soaking my hair. The icy water ran down my body in rivulets, pooling on the bathroom carpet. He didn't stop until I was thoroughly drenched and shivering.

'You mean nothing to the Party,' he said coldly. 'And when you've been tortured enough you'll confess to anything. Everything.'

I stayed silent, internalising the fear and alienation of being in Nikolaja's situation.

'You have no friends, no allies. No one to speak up for you.'

Cameron continued in that vein for several minutes. Tears welled in my eyes and I lowered my head meekly as he led me back down the hall to the makeup room. In my mind I ran through all the things Nikolaja had suffered up to this point in the story: forced exercise, sensory deprivation, riding the wooden horse, back and genital whipping, caning, bastinado . . . Nikolaja was one stubborn girl; I'd have given in long before all that.

Then he said something about my dead father, the traitor, and I found the hook I needed to stay defiant. Because if Nikolaja was a spy, then her father was too. I had a very clear image in my head: signing the confession would be equivalent to writing: *My father was a traitor.*

When they were ready for me, I was so much in Nikolaja's head that I didn't see the familiar faces of friends and fellow actors. I saw The Enemy. There were eight of them there, surrounding me and looking down on me. I was thoroughly intimidated. Naked, handcuffed, cold and wet. Terrified. I didn't have to fake anything.

Having a gun held to your head is an indescribable experience. Scary even when you know it's not real. My heart hammered painfully in my chest and the adrenalin overload made me feel weightless. I whispered frantically, 'Please don't kill me,' again and again. Tormans Elefernus, who played the Soviet counsellor, said afterwards that he was afraid I was going to break down for real.

The scene is in slow motion in the film and that's exactly how I experienced it. I swear I heard the friction of the counsellor's finger on the trigger as he pulled it. And the empty CLICK! seemed like an explosion. I came undone.

It was so real for me. The fear, the exhilaration, the background worry that it could all go horribly wrong . . . I collapsed on the floor, sobbing and shaking uncontrollably, babbling that I'd sign anything. Someone handed me a pen and I managed an illegible scrawl on the paper with a violently trembling hand as waves of cathartic tears overwhelmed me.

17. CAMARADERIE OF SUFFERING

After lunch, it was time to be tortured. Kateřina, Jana and I sat together in the prison cell while the crew set up the dungeon on the other side of the partition. My Czech had improved somewhat, but the complicated declensions and conjugations still made it impossible to convey even the simplest ideas. But we managed to entertain ourselves in spite of the language barrier. Reduced to pointing at things and naming them in a me-Tarzan-you-Jane way, we made a game out of it.

'*Co je slovo?*' I asked, pointing at the antique typewriter. (What is word?)

'*Psací stroj*,' Kateřina said.

I mangled the word trying to repeat it.

'*Anglicky?*' Jana asked. (In English?)

'Typewriter.'

They managed better than I had and we moved on to the next word.

'Prison,' I said, indicating the cell.

'*Vězení*,' Jana supplied in Czech.

Kateřina rubbed her bottom. '*To bolí*,' she said ruefully.

'It hurts,' I agreed.

Jana mimed swinging a cane.

'*Rákoskou!*' I said triumphantly. A word I knew!

Kateřina countered with '*Der Rohrstock*.' She also spoke German, so when Czech and English failed us we tried it instead, creating our own pidgin language. A couple of people overheard our linguistic soup and shook their heads, grinning. Soon we'd have to be political prisoners, but for now we were playing like kids.

We also had fun with my Czech phrasebook. Lonely Planet ones are the best. They have a special section on 'romance' that tells you how to say useful things like 'Please (don't) stop!', 'I'd like us to stay friends' and 'I'm sorry, I can't get it up'. I love the image of a man fumbling for the phrasebook mid-thrust to say, 'I hope you've been tested for sexual diseases.'

Our language games came to an end when the torture chamber was ready for its first victim. It's one of the most interesting sequences in any Lupus film. One by one each prisoner suffers some creative punishment. Then one signs the confession. The remaining victims suffer different punishments until another one breaks. And so on. Nikolaja is the last one. At the end of the sequence there are three confessions signed and one unsigned.

The torture scenes were inventive and most of them were firsts for me. For one, they shackled my wrists and strung me up to expose my back for a whipping. I overheard Zbyšek asking Cameron, 'How hard should he beat her?'

Cameron inspected the thin strap and said, 'As hard as he can,' he said. 'She'd be disappointed with anything less.'

I thought I would faint. All these men were discussing what to do with me and how to treat me. What they decided would happen. It might not have been Nikolaja's fantasy, but it was certainly mine.

There's a special freedom in being able to scream at the top of your lungs. But our cries were ignored. Our suffering meant nothing. And why should it? They didn't actually expect us to give them any information; this was about breaking us.

Throughout the tortures I was lost in the role. But as soon as Zbyšek yelled 'Cut!' I was myself again, comforted and released by the same people who'd strung me up and beaten me. It's only five strokes, but you're meant to imagine it lasting as long as the canings had. The other girls admired my marks and we giggled together. Then it was Kateřina's turn.

It was peculiarly intimate – a camaraderie of suffering. And while Kateřina was beaten, Jana and I held each other's hands for comfort. When it was over, we admired Kateřina's marks and then it was Jana's turn. Then Alexandra's. Then mine again. In between scenes we'd huddle together and wait to see who was called in next.

During the torments, something strange happened. I found my anxiety fading. I've heard that victims of real torture can sometimes rise above the pain. Each successive scene was painful and scary, but as time passed I seemed to draw the energy and power away from my tormentors and make it my own. I felt empowered rather than weakened. I transcended the suffering. I was honestly disappointed when it was over.

When we'd all confessed to being spies, we were free to go. My entire body ached. Kateřina and Jana were in a similar state. Our bottoms hurt from the caning the day before. Our wrists and ankles were bruised and chafed from the rough iron shackles and the hard wooden plank we'd been bound to. I had some peculiar bow-tie-shaped marks on my back from the strap. And, like warriors, we proudly showed off our victory scars. We had survived. I saved the cane they broke on my feet, a souvenir of one of my scariest moments.

As always, there was that familiar sadness when it was all over. Back to life, back to reality. My limits had been pushed further than ever before – physically and psychologically. I couldn't have taken any more abuse, but I still didn't want it to be over.

I wrote another article for the Lupus website, called 'Tales from the Dark Side'. The last line was, 'If Lupus ever makes a film set in a madhouse, I can guess who they'll call . . .'

A year later those words would come back to haunt me.

Hiya. R U the REAL Niki or just someone using her handle for a better impact?

Doppelganger, UK

18. BEING NIKI FLYNN

It's something I never could have predicted – that people would doubt I was me. Of course, if someone appeared in a chat room claiming to be Nicole Kidman you'd be suspicious. But I'm not a Hollywood movie star. I'm just a kinky girl who's lucky enough to be able to do what she loves.

It's an interesting exercise trying to prove you're you. How do you do it? I know lots of things about 'Niki Flynn' that no one else does. I know her real name for a start. I also know her address, her favourite colour and a million other things. But none of it counts as proof. Who'd believe me anyway? It's truly bizarre to be confronted with the accusation that you're an impostor. Of yourself.

The first time I got a message asking if I was the 'real' Niki Flynn I thought it was a wind-up. But the second one made me realise that people were serious. Baffled, I asked the members of one of the spanking forums what it was all about. They said it was just hard for someone to grasp the idea that there are real people behind these famous bottoms. They think we do it for the money and the only reason we post on forums is to promote our videos. Well, fair enough. *I* know that's not the case, but people who haven't met me have no way of knowing.

A few months later I joined a German forum and was lured into the chat room despite my protests that my German wasn't very good. 'We speak your language too,' my correspondent assured me.

Well, as soon as I went in, someone called Gustav asked if I was really 'the' Niki Flynn. I was flattered, but I had that Twilight Zone feeling again. How do you answer that? 'Yes, I'm *the* one and only, world-renowned famous movie star . . .' It's crazy!

One of the girls in the chat room had said she spoke English, but not well. So I was using very simple English with her, and she was using very simple German with me.

'This is not the English that Niki Flynn speaks,' Gustav wrote. 'You're obviously not a native English speaker.'

I had no answer for that.

'What's your US address?' he demanded. 'How would you write it on an envelope?'

When I declined to broadcast that information in the chat room he declared it was proof that I was an impostor.

Finally, he asked me a couple of spanking-related questions and when the answers matched what he'd read about me elsewhere he said, 'You've simply studied the David Pierson interview.' So if you throw me in the river and I don't drown . . . I'm a witch. I just didn't know what to say.

Someone on my Yahoo group suggested I change my name and vehemently deny being me. If I never admitted it, people might believe me. I was tempted.

Of course, the more obvious hazard of notoriety is *being* recognised. That's not really a problem in a kinky venue, but there are times when I'm at the gym or in an airport and catch someone staring at me. My first paranoid thought is that they're trying to decide whether I'm really the spanking model I look so much like.

I was in London once with Cameron and we decided to see if they had any of my videos in the Soho sex shops. UK Customs and Excise frown on importing Lupus videos into the UK, but pirate copies abound. It's a big problem for the maker, whose products are freely available everywhere else in the EU. But the ultimate irony is that I'd never have seen the films in the first place if they hadn't been pirated. I'd never have asked to be in one and I might never have become a spanking model at all. It's kind of poetic.

Even though they were pirate copies, it was still exciting to see my movies on the shelves. We found them in three shops that specialise in spanking porn. One customer was looking at the

Lupus videos when we came in. I don't know if he recognised me or if he simply overheard our conversation, but he picked up the DVD of *Exchange Student* and looked over at me as if to compare.

The man behind the till was watching. Finally he asked, 'Are you Niki Flynn?'

It was all I could do not to squeal with delight. *I've made it*, I thought. *I'm a star!*

Occasionally I Google my name to see what comes up. One day I was surprised to see a new website with the same name and spelling as me: niki-flynn.com. I followed the link to an Australian site advertising 'Niki Flynn' designer jeans! Their exclusive 'drive-by' range featured jeans that had been shot with a .45 magnum revolver. I *had* to have a pair.

I wrote to the address on the site and asked where I could buy them. The lady who replied was delighted that I had the same name as the jeans and she asked me to tell her about myself. She even offered me a 25 per cent discount on a pair of jeans.

I could just imagine the company getting emails asking if the jeans were cane-proof, so I felt I ought to warn her. I couldn't believe they hadn't done a search on the name before registering the site. Surely they wondered why nikiflynn.com without the hyphen was already taken.

I wrote back with a discreet description of who I was and what I did. I suggested that she Google the name herself. I fear it was a nasty shock; she never responded.

(drama school, age 18)

Today I had the most amazing experience. We've been doing lots of improv and roleplay to learn how to get in touch with emotional parts of ourselves. Mr Wynn gives us a scenario and tells us who we are. Then we just go with it. You can tap into some really primal stuff. Sometimes it's painful, but it's freeing to be so open, so raw. It's like letting something in.

This one involved the whole class – all twenty of us. Mr Wynn split us into two groups and sent us to opposite sides of the stage. My group stood in the wings stage-left while he went to talk to the first group. All we could hear were low murmurs. He was with them for a long time – nearly ten minutes. We looked around at each other, wondering what was being said and what he was about to spring on us. Finally, he came to my group.

'For the past year you have all been prisoners of war,' he said softly. 'And terrible things have been done to you in the internment camp.'

I glanced at Daniel beside me. He looked away. Some of the others shifted uncomfortably.

Mr Wynn told us to think about what we'd been through, the abuse we'd suffered and the terror and pain that had become our daily existence.

I looked at the floor, feeling the chill in the room, trying to imagine what had happened to us. I closed my eyes and let his voice guide me into a dark cave. No one knew what I was seeing in my cave and I didn't know what anyone else was seeing in theirs. I felt Daniel move closer to me.

'You haven't seen your friends or family since you were captured,' said Mr Wynn. 'And you don't know if they're alive or dead.'

One of the girls started crying at that and I pressed closer to Daniel, not wanting to be infected by her grief. I felt myself building walls inside, just as I had as a child. I huddled into myself, swallowing my tears.

'Now the camp has been liberated. And you're free. You're on a train heading back to your village.'

His voice became the gentle rocking of a train taking us home to an uncertain future. The air felt stagnant.

'We're here,' he said in a whisper. 'It's time to step off the train.'

Slowly I opened my eyes. We had inched closer and closer until we were all cowering together. No one was crying now. I looked around cautiously at the others, but none of us wanted to make eye contact. We didn't even look at the villagers, who were standing on the platform a few feet away.

I convinced myself we weren't really free, that it was all just a cruel trick. I felt frightened and mistrustful, locked inside my pain. Unreachable. I didn't want to see anyone I knew. The fear of them knowing what had happened to me was greater than my fear of being sent back. I was ashamed.

The deeper I allowed myself to sink into the emotional pain, the stronger the feelings grew. I felt profoundly alone.

The stage was silent. Nobody moved. The two groups stood facing each other for several minutes. Finally one of the villagers stepped forward and reached out to one of the prisoners. Out of the corner of my eye I saw them embrace and then slowly the others followed suit.

All at once I was blinded with tears. I couldn't see the girl who gathered me in her arms. I stood stiffly, resisting, but she didn't let go. That broke me. I clung to her, a beautiful pale blur whose silky hair smelled like rosewater, like solace. Like home.

19. SHADOW LANE

Twice a year, enthusiasts from all over the US (and a few other countries) gather for a weekend of spanking and socialising. The parties are organised by Tony Elka and Eve Howard, who run Shadow Lane, a spanking film company with the tagline 'the romance of discipline'. Picture the scene: a hotel descended on by spankos. Adults in school uniform in the lobby, bright-red bottoms by the pool, the sound of smacking coming from nearly every room . . .

This was the last party to be held at the Riviera Hotel in Palm Springs, California. Elvis and Frank Sinatra had performed there. It was a gorgeous sunny retreat – perfect for a long weekend of playing and partying.

The party's location changes, but the programme stays the same. On Friday night there's a vendors' fair, where toymakers and video producers sell their products. And on Saturday there's a buffet dinner and dancing. People mingle and play and exchange room numbers and invitations to private parties, which is where most of the real action happens. I can't imagine what the vanilla guests make of it.

It's the spanko equivalent of a swingers' club, except that there's no sex. Well, some people probably have sex, but only in private. The vast majority of play takes place in rooms filled with people and public sexual play is frowned upon.

Not everyone is lucky enough to have a kinky partner and the freedom to play at home. For them parties offer the ultimate kinky getaway, a chance to cram as much play as possible into the weekend. There's a lot of partner-swapping and lap-hopping. I've seen women go straight from one man's lap to another's for more spanking. There are strict etiquette rules about negotiating play and anyone who violates limits is given the boot. It's a place where spankos can let themselves go and indulge their fetish in a totally safe environment.

Cameron and I were a little jet-lagged, but we didn't let that spoil our fun. I was surprised that so many people knew who I was. Shadow Lane videos are at the softer end of the spectrum, and I didn't expect many Lupus fans to be there. They peppered me with the usual questions: was it fake? Were the Czech girls coerced? It's amazing how far such rumours reach.

People were already playing in the main room and the vendor fair offered plenty of excuses. Naturally, you have to try out a toy before deciding to buy it and guinea pigs aren't hard to find. The London Tanner is renowned in the Scene for his quality leather straps. He makes everything himself, from authentic Scottish tawses to replica prison straps. Tops love them; bottoms love to hate them. I found myself bent over his table while Cameron tested implements on my bottom. Everyone was watching. Ah, the exhibitionistic bliss!

You can never have too many toys. Even though Cameron has a substantial arsenal, we buy something new at every party. Transporting them is always an adventure, especially when canes are involved. Their length is inconvenient, so you have to be creative. Next time you see a convention of shifty-eyed golfers and fishermen, ask yourself whether those cases really contain clubs and fly rods.

One guy I know put his entire collection of toys in an architectural blueprints tube, but failed to seal it properly. He dropped it in the airport and implements went everywhere. I'm sure the security guys have seen it all, but I still shudder at the prospect of my suitcase bursting open as the baggage handlers hurl it onto the trolley, sending canes and paddles clattering across the tarmac.

Nearly every spanko has some embarrassing story to tell. There's the Canadian couple who forgot to put their toys away before leaving the hotel room. They returned to find the room made up and all the toys neatly lined up in a row at the foot of the bed. Then there's Debbie, who failed to cancel the window cleaner on the day she'd scheduled a play session with her boyfriend. Oops!

And there are countless stories of what tradesmen have seen. My friend Marie put all her boyfriend's kinky toys in the bottom of a chest of drawers when she moved house. The clumsy removal men tilted it the wrong way as they lifted it. The drawer slid out and *voila!* She was clever enough to shrug nonchalantly and let them assume she was the domme. They worked quickly after that.

I used to worry about people seeing the brass dance pole in the middle of our bedroom, but, oddly enough, most of the time they walk right past it without noticing it. It's hard to miss the school desk and gym horse in the attic, though. And a clever person might spot the bolts and hooks Cameron has installed for attaching ropes to the beams. Not that they'd ever say anything.

My favourite scene of the weekend was a private lesson from my friend Lee, a professional ballet dancer. I'd had lessons as a little girl, but I couldn't stick with it. That D word again. Ballet is all about discipline.

I'd met Lee and her husband Sergei on a spanking forum and we'd been corresponding for months. This was our first face-to-face meeting. Lee was strict and elegant, with impeccable posture. The quintessential ballet mistress. You couldn't mistake her for anything else.

Sergei played accompanist, choosing selections of music on his laptop while Cameron took pictures to send them afterwards as a memento. Lee had me doing pliés and relevés, all the while correcting my posture and totting up the numbers when I screwed up.

'Boneless arms,' she instructed. 'Don't sickle your feet. Tuck your bottom in.'

I was extremely self-conscious at first, a grown-up in a child's class. But I trusted Lee not to humiliate me. She was inflicting very advanced stuff on me and I succumbed to the vulnerability of being completely out of my depth. The authenticity of her teaching got to me and I tuned the men out. The hotel room vanished and I was in the ballet studio alone with Lee.

At the end of the lesson she caned me for all the mistakes I'd made. She placed me with my hands on the bed, my back parallel to the floor and my head up. She was very precise about the posture she wanted. I was allowed to kick and squirm (staying still is not an option for me!), but I had to resume the position immediately. Maintaining posture and elegance despite the pain is crucial in ballet. I did my best to make her proud.

It was a great experience for me. A satisfying roleplay that wasn't really a roleplay at all. My bottom was very tender by the end of the scene. I actually learned a lot about ballet too, though my legs were so sore from stretching in unfamiliar ways that it hurt to walk the next day. I felt taller, like I'd been on a rack in a mediæval dungeon. But I loved my tormentress. I only wished she'd conducted our little 'class' in French.

I got some strange looks from vanilla guests as I slipped through the corridors in my leotard, tights and ballet slippers. Poor things. As if the school uniforms and smacking weren't weird enough.

Unfortunately, my play that weekend was limited. I had to take care of what Cameron calls 'the Flynn-bottom'. I'd arranged to shoot with the Denver-based company RealSpankings a week after the party, so I couldn't afford to have marks.

You can always tell the newbies by their fabulous welts and bruises. But an experienced bottom is harder to mark. Repeated spanking toughens the capillaries so that bruising diminishes over time.

Most players cherish marks. They're a reminder of the scene until they fade. It's delicious to be out in public, sitting gingerly and no one the wiser. Shifting deliberately just to reawaken the soft ache and remember how those bruises got there.

But a movie shoot demands a pristine bottom at the start. I didn't want to disappoint the viewers, so I kept my play light. One of the hazards of the business.

Hey Niki Flynn,

You like uniforms, do you? I wonder if my dress blues can be dusted off after 25 years of languishing in a packing box. I have a sword too – a nice long flat cold-steel sword. Ever been spanked with the flat of a sword, girl?

I want to do a scene with you. You are a girl in a sailors' waterfront place, combination barmaid and available-for-a-price girl. I'm a rough sailor, back in port after, oh – a season or two at sea. I'm in my dungarees, watch cap and peacoat. I arrange with the owner to take you in the back. When we get to the room you start to undress and flirt. But I grab you and put you over my knee and spank you hard. You continue to flirt. I strip you and throw you on the bed, tying you down with your stockings. Then I take off my broad leather belt. It's OK for you to scream now!

Billy the China Fleet Gob, Kowloon

20. THE CONSPIRACY

'Get your fucking hands off me!'
Two teachers and a prefect try to restrain me, but I've had enough of this place. RS Institute. Ha! I'm not putting on their stupid uniform. I'm outta here! But the three women drag me back into the room and hold me down on the couch. I fight back, screaming and cursing.

Mr Daniels arrives, astonished at the commotion. 'What is going on here?' he demands.

The women try to explain that I'm the new arrival. 'And she is trouble!' Ms Burns adds.

Mr Daniels hauls me up on my feet and snarls, 'Listen, it's either get along or get spanked. You understand?'

I spit in his face. Now the gloves are off.

The four of them wrestle me to the floor face-down and Mr Daniels tells me I've just made it much worse for myself. He plants his knee against the back of my neck, pinning me to the floor. Immobilised, I can only gasp and pant, resisting feebly as he cuts my clothing away with a pair of scissors. My strength is waning, but not my pride. I refuse to go down without a fight. I continue to struggle as he bares my bottom, snipping away the flimsy thong and giving me a hard spanking that makes my eyes water.

He's just made a serious enemy. And when I get my chance I intend to make him pay.

It was supposed to be a kidnapping in an old warehouse. Just 'Coach' Daniels and me. We'd talked via email and both of us were really excited about the idea. Coach had spent ten years in the US Marine Corps; hard resistance play was one of his specialities. We brainstormed about the scene, wondering how edgy the producers would let us get.

All this was arranged before the Shadow Lane party. But a few days before Cameron and I left for California I got an email from Lady D at RealSpankings. The kidnapping was off. Perhaps the idea was too much for them after all. Instead, she proposed a slumber party with four girls. RS owns several websites, some devoted to individual girls. She wanted to bring some of those girls in for a kind of 'all-stars' movie. I said that was fine, though I felt cheated out of my kidnapping. I packed my pyjamas and we left for the States.

After the party we set off on the week-long road trip to Denver. First we stopped at Zion National Park for a five-mile hike up the canyon wall to Angel's Landing. It was an intimidating trail with gruelling switchbacks and dizzying narrow ridges. But the fairy-tale view from the top was worth all the pain and anxiety. There's always a sense of achievement at the end of a hike like that. Then you remember that you still have to get back down. Our feet were sore and blistered by the time we reached the bottom. Cameron drove us to our motel, where we limped inside and collapsed.

By morning, we were ready for the next national park. We spent the day at Bryce Canyon exploring the strange rock formations. The sandstone spires and columns make a landscape of breathtaking alien beauty. We got lost among the hoodoos and had to ration our water until we found the path again.

That night I got a message on my phone from Lady D. She'd lost the location for the slumber party.

I rolled my eyes, growing more and more frustrated. I imagined the worst when we got to Denver: lame apologies for having wasted my time and maybe a token fee for my trouble. I didn't expect any recompense for all the play I'd missed out on at the party in saving my bottom for them. The new idea was simply to do some clips for the RS website.

I made a face. 'If I'd known they wanted me to come all this way just for some stupid clips I'd have said no thanks!'

Ah, well. The road trip was fabulous. At Arches we found a secluded spot and Cameron convinced me to strip off for some nude photos. The Utah sun beat down on me as I posed for him, keeping one eye peeled for hikers.

I found a rocky outcrop that formed a natural stage and I abandoned all my inhibitions. I curved my body into a backbend, echoing the line of the sandstone arch above me. I felt exuberant. Free and wild. I danced to the music of the wind as it shook the dry limbs of the desert trees.

It took me several minutes to notice that I was being watched. The man smiled broadly when he realised I'd seen him. I hurriedly ducked behind a rock and he went on his way, still smiling.

'You certainly made his day.' Cameron laughed.

'What if he's off to report me to the park ranger?' I scampered down from my stage and dusted myself off, shaking the grit out of my clothes as I got dressed.

'Oh, he won't report you.'

'Probably not, but next time we might not be so lucky.'

One male voyeur I could handle, but I wasn't keen to traumatise a busload of schoolchildren.

As we set off for Canyonlands the next day my phone bleeped. Sure enough, there was another change of plans. Now, however, things were looking up. The clips were off; they'd written a storyline for a proper movie instead. I would be the new arrival at the RS Institute, a reformatory alternative to prison. And I would be a Very Bad Girl Indeed. The worst arrival they'd ever had to deal with. That sounded great to me and I especially liked the forced stripping scene outlined in the message.

The rest of the story was equally promising. After the stripping and a hard hand-spanking from Mr Daniels, I befriend Bailey, the resident good girl. I promptly sneak a bottle of alcohol into her dorm room and we get caught by Mr Daniels and caned. In the next scene Mr Daniels berates Ms Burns in front of the class (four of us, including RS regulars Kailee and Brandi) before insisting that she give Bailey and me a hard strapping for cheating. She'd left us alone in the classroom, you see. Naughty, naughty.

Ms Burns isn't at all pleased at having her authority undermined in front of her class. And Miss Baker, another teacher, is resentful at being reprimanded for leaving the premises for personal reasons. Both teachers are tired of the tyrannical Mr Daniels, but Ms Burns has a plan – the eponymous conspiracy. They hold a meeting and invite the four of us along. She and Miss Baker will plant some dubious photos in Mr Daniels's office if we'll make corroborating complaints of sexual harassment. When he's gone, the school can go back to normal. The students are all on board, even sweet little Bailey.

The camera takes in our determined faces before panning along the wall to reveal a hidden webcam. Cut to Mr Daniels, shaking his head as he watches the video of our mutinous assembly. I bet you can't guess what he offers in lieu of expulsion.

'This is great!' I said to Cameron.

He agreed. 'Six girls paddled at the end? That will be intense.'

RS was renowned for its severe school paddlings. I'd seen their early work – schoolgirls and cheerleaders grabbing their ankles for the board and then kneeling facing the wall with their skirts up, bullseye bruises on their bottoms. Six of us lined up like that would be quite a spectacle.

At Canyonlands we hiked to the edge of a cliff for an awe-inspiring view over the vast gorge. It was completely silent and still, not a breath of wind. We could have been the only people in the world.

'There's no one here,' Cameron said. 'And this is a stunning location for some photography.'

I knew what he meant. I was nervous about it, but I couldn't argue. A naked girl in front of that yawning chasm would be a striking image.

I undressed behind a boulder and crept to the edge of the overlook. I'm not usually afraid of heights, but peering down into that abyss was enough to make me light-headed. Keeping a respectful distance from the crumbling stone at the edge, I adopted some shy, self-conscious poses, paranoid about someone happening on our little shoot.

'We're not doing anything wrong,' Cameron assured me. 'We're just taking some artsy photos.'

I began to relax and let myself go as I had the day before. So what if some prissy schoolmarm happened upon us? Big deal. I was a child of nature, celebrating the beauty of the world.

As I grew more confident, Cameron suggested I try some ballet poses. I did my best to remember everything Lee had taught me at Shadow Lane, focusing on lines and balance. The picture I'm proudest of is a back view of me near the edge of the cliff. My feet are in first position, my arms held gracefully over my head. And spread out before me is the immense canyon, stretching into eternity. (I emailed it to Lee that night and was delighted when she praised my posture.)

A minute later we heard the unmistakable crunch of hiking boots on gravel. I scurried back to my boulder just as an elderly lady appeared on the path to the overlook. I didn't waste time putting on my bra and panties; I just threw my shirt and shorts on over my dusty body.

In the distance I heard Cameron asking if she wouldn't mind hanging back for a minute. 'My girlfriend is using the ladies' room,' he explained politely.

Behind my rock, I blushed.

When we arrived in Denver I immediately succumbed to the altitude sickness that affects most first-time visitors. It wouldn't make much difference with me, though. I'd be sick in the morning anyway.

When my phone bleeped that night we exchanged a weary look.

'I don't even want to know,' I groaned.

Cameron read the message. 'No, it's not bad,' he said. 'She wants to change what you're getting up to with Bailey in her dorm room.'

'Smuggled booze isn't bad enough? What does she want me to do instead?'

He grinned. 'Have sex with her.'

'*What?*'

'She says, "Nothing graphic, don't worry. The lights will be out and Bailey will just moan and gasp. Then Coach will burst in and turn on the lights and discover you under the blanket."'

I had to laugh. It sounded innocent enough. 'That's fine,' I said. 'I just hope I like this Bailey girl.'

It's always scary going into an established 'family'. You're guaranteed to feel like an outsider. But the RS crew were friendly and welcoming and they made Cameron and me feel right at home.

We shot the intake scene first, where prefect Kailee explains the rules to me. A striking girl with pale skin and dark hair, Kailee was one of the most popular RS girls. I was intimidated about meeting so many famous spanking models until someone told me that they were just as intimidated about meeting *me*! It's impossible to have any perspective on your public persona.

Kailee told me she hated dialogue, especially improv. Still, she was a lot better than I was. All I did was curse like a sailor. Guys told me later that the movie needed a mouth-soaping scene.

Then came the dramatic stripping. Fortunately, they provided the disposable costume. Normally I'd have come equipped with something of my own, but I didn't have enough notice. The synopsis had said that Coach would cut off my clothes with scissors. What he did was even better. He cut a slit in the bottom of my shirt and then ripped it the rest of the way up. I'd never realised how sexy the sound of tearing fabric could be.

Naked, spanked, exhausted and (temporarily) humbled, I was delivered into the care of Miss Baker, who led me away.

It was a successful first scene. I recovered the pearl earring I'd lost in my struggles. I had carpet burns on my legs and belly. Ms Burns had left livid nail marks on my arms. And my vocal cords were shredded from screaming. The thin dry air of the mile-high city had no pity for me and I simply couldn't stop coughing. It went on so long it became embarrassing. Lady D gave me some cough drops, which helped while I was sucking on them. I wondered if I'd be able to talk at all without them. No one seemed too bothered, though.

'No problem,' Lady D said. 'Just take your time and we'll start again when you're ready. We need to wait for Bailey anyway.'

Ah yes, Bailey. My lesbian lover. I was nervous again.

I went to put on the RS uniform and Lady D recruited Cameron to help set up the schoolroom. No one else could reach the overhead light bulbs.

Eventually, after a whole roll of cough drops and about a gallon of water, I was able to talk. And just in time. Bailey had arrived.

My co-star looked every inch the fresh-faced girl next door. Her innocence is part of her charm and her fans cherish her peachy complexion and freckles. She was fairly new to the world of spanking films. So far she'd only done website clips; this was her first movie. Fortunately, she was nervous too.

'Apparently we have a love scene,' I said.

'So I gather. I only found out about it this morning. Lady D said, "Oh, by the way, you're doing a love scene with Niki."'

We shared a laugh over that. Then Coach sobered us up by showing us the cane he'd be using after breaking up our little tryst.

Bailey shuddered. 'I really hate the cane.'

'But it's so much classier than the paddle,' I insisted. 'The board's the one that really scares me.'

When it was time for our big scene, Bailey and I stripped off our clothes and climbed into bed together. Even though I'd just spent two days dancing naked in national parks, it was still embarrassing. Our discarded pyjamas lay on the floor beside the bed. Bailey lay on her back and I curled up beside her. The urge to tickle all that exposed pink flesh was strong, but I managed to resist. I didn't fancy an inadvertent knee in the face. We both felt awkward and silly, though we knew the viewers would love it.

'You'll have to be the bratty one,' Bailey told me. She's a lifestyle submissive, so rebellion isn't easy for her.

I'm the complete opposite. I like to submit because my character has been coerced or forced – or because it's a well-deserved punishment. But I don't have the deep desire to please that characterises a truly submissive nature. I consider myself a bottom, but not a submissive. It's a subtle distinction, but an important one.

As for being bratty, I adore getting to say and do the outrageous things I never did when I was in school. On film I get to be the bad girl I never was.

When Lady D told Bailey to make some sexual noises, her efforts were laughably unconvincing. For once I had the easier role.

'Come on, Bailey,' said Lady D. 'You know the noises I mean!'

The cast and crew offered their own interpretations of hot girl-girl porno sound effects. From my position under the covers, it sounded like an orgy. There was no way I'd be able to keep a straight face. Not that it mattered; the camera couldn't *see* my face.

The lights went out and we started the scene. Bailey writhed under the blanket, moaning and gasping in the throes of violent ecstasy.

Suddenly a door opened and light flooded the room. I flattened myself out beside Bailey and listened to the exchange.

'Who is in there with you, Bailey?'

'Um . . .'

I heard footsteps and then the blanket was whipped off, exposing two naked girls cowering together.

Mr Daniels was appalled. 'This is not good!' (That line's a Coach classic; he says it a *lot*.) 'I'm doing night checks and this is what I find? You having sex with another girl? *Not good!*'

'We weren't having sex!' I acted outraged and looked to Bailey for confirmation. No help there; she looked petrified.

'Judging by the sounds coming out of her little mouth, you were having sex!'

'Well, get your mind out of the gutter, man,' I retorted.

Bailey's 'Oh, shit!' expression was priceless.

Mr Daniels grabbed my hair and told me I was really in for it. He dragged us out of bed and told Bailey to assume the position first. She would get six strokes; I would get twice that.

Earlier, Lady D had asked us how many strokes we should get. Bailey's pale skin marked dramatically, so they didn't want to give her too much. She still had a hard strapping and a paddling to look forward to. But a light caning for such a serious infraction would look lame on film. Cameron solved the problem with the helpful suggestion that I get double whatever Bailey got, as I was the instigator.

'Just doing my job,' he told me with a shrug.

Boyfriends on set have a bad reputation with some companies. Apparently they can get overprotective. Not Cameron.

Bailey obediently placed her hands on the bed and bent over while I stood off to the side, forced to watch. I hate going last. Having to watch someone else get it first, knowing that you're next, increases the anxiety tenfold.

The cane rose and fell while Bailey cried out in pain. By the end of the six strokes, her face was streaming with tears. Bailey's good at crying.

I took my twelve with much yelping and kicking while Mr Daniels told Bailey this was what she could expect if she associated with 'girls like this'. Me? The bad influence? *If only they could see Goody Two Shoes now*, I thought.

21. DEAD PUPPIES

The crew took half an hour to set up the final scene. They'd never filmed a mass paddling before and the room was barely wide enough to get us all in shot. While they fiddled with the equipment and discussed shooting angles, we psyched ourselves up for the scene. We were determined to cry.

Someone asked, 'What makes you cry?'

'Dead puppies,' I said.

'Oh, that's too sad!'

'Makes you cry, though.'

'That song from *Titanic*,' someone else offered.

I imagined Kate Winslet croaking, 'Jack, there's a boat,' and my eyes blurred with tears.

And on it went, with everyone offering sad songs or movie lines or images to get us to the brink of tears. Hey, man, we're serious actors!

Ms Burns was strategically placed at the head of the line. 'I always cry,' she said. 'Maybe that will help.'

We formed a line to her right. Ms Burns, Brandi, me, Bailey, Kailee and Miss Baker. One camera shot us from behind while a handheld in front of us showed our nervous faces. Really, Ms Burns should have gone last for dramatic effect. She was the instigator of the conspiracy, after all.

'Dead puppies, dead puppies,' we chanted softly, earning a weird look from the cameraman. A satanic rite? Hogwarts spell? No, just six spanking models trying to muster tears.

The cameras rolled. The four students and two teachers listened with apprehension while Mr Daniels told us how foolish we'd been. Our sedition, he said, would be severely dealt with. He paced along the line like a sadistic sergeant-major, smacking a fearsome school paddle against his hand. Lest we forget what we were about to receive.

This particular paddle was special: a fan had made it for the RS studio. It was honey-coloured maple, about a foot long, four inches wide and three-eighths of an inch thick. Not as ferocious as a fraternity paddle, but it would still hurt plenty.

He told us to bend over and raise our skirts, which we did with trembling hands. Tears were already rolling down Kailee's face. One by one he took our panties down.

'I hope this isn't sexual harassment, Ms Burns,' he said sarcastically as he exposed her bottom. 'Now take one step back.'

She obeyed and I held my breath as I waited for the first stroke. It's hard enough to watch someone else get punished knowing you're next, but it's truly cruel when you can only *hear* it. The first crack of the paddle made me jump and Ms Burns was in tears instantly, barely able to choke out 'One, sir'. Listening to the ten hard swats took me right back to high school, where I used to listen with fear and morbid curiosity to the punishments down the hall.

Contrary to the way it's portrayed in CP films, the paddle was never given on the bare – not at my school, anyway. Never even on the panties. And it was never more than a couple of swats. 'Pops', we called it. And it was a joke. Certainly nothing anyone feared and, judging by the recidivists, no deterrent. But while most CP films claim to strive for authenticity, what they really want to create is the *illusion* of authenticity. It is a fantasy, after all. Two light 'pops' over clothes would not make a compelling movie.

'Ten, sir,' sobbed Ms Burns.

'Step back in line.'

Still crying, she shuffled back to her place. It was Brandi's turn. The poor girl had the flu that day, but Coach didn't cut her any slack. There would be time to praise her dedication when the scene was over. Ten times the paddle slammed into her bottom while she yelped and cried and counted, putting me more and more on edge.

Before I knew it, it was my turn. I took a step back and placed my hands on my knees. The paddle touched my bottom, which was already tender from the earlier scenes. It raised up and smacked into me with shocking force. Unlike the cane, you feel the impact of a paddle instantly. It's like sitting on a hot stove. (Not that I've actually done that.)

I was used to the sting of the cane, but I didn't get paddled often on film or in private. My bottom was ablaze with pain. It was impossible to think of anything else. Cameron told me afterwards that he'd never seen a paddle used that hard before. Still, I managed to count each stroke, trying to ignore the cameraman in front of me.

I returned to my place in the line, shaken and crying. But I couldn't feel relief yet. We were only halfway there; three more girls had their turns coming.

Bailey sobbed and cried out loudly, making me flinch at each stroke. I was glad to know she was kinky because she truly seemed to be hating every minute of it. Like me, she hates the cause and loves the effect. I counted silently with her to number eight, but Bailey was in so much distress she counted nine.

Mr Daniels waited until she realised her mistake and corrected herself. 'Eight, sir!'

It's a common ploy of bratty bottoms to miscount and hope the top won't notice. It always earns you extra if you get caught. However, with Bailey it had been an honest mistake, and Mr Daniels didn't give her an extra stroke for it.

I closed my eyes in vicarious relief as the paddle struck home again and she counted the proper number nine. There was a pause and for a moment I worried that the extra stroke was coming after all. But instead, Mr Daniels decided she'd had enough and told her, 'Your bottom's done. Sorry. Get back in line.'

Sniffling, she moved back to her place beside me and I reached for her hand, giving her a comforting sisterly squeeze.

Kailee was tough and stoic. She'd been crying before the paddling started, but now she was determined not to show any weakness. Mr Daniels commented that she was a girl who knew how to take a paddling. *Teacher's pet*, I thought. *Just wait till the sequel*.

Miss Baker was the one I really felt sorry for. I would have been near panic after listening to the other five take their swats first. She endured it bravely, crying and counting. But again, rather than risk damage, Mr Daniels stopped early, sparing her the last two strokes.

Mr Daniels told us all to kneel with our skirts up and our arms behind our backs, the traditional RS 'time-out' position. Then he stepped back to admire his handiwork: a row of severely punished bottoms on display, each sporting the paddle's distinctive bullseye bruises. Some were marked more than others. Ms Burns's bottom was the most dramatic, but Bailey's and Miss Baker's were close behind.

'Great job, everyone!' Lady D said.

But Bailey was miffed. 'It was only one more stroke,' she pouted to Coach. 'You shouldn't have stopped. You made me feel like a wimp.'

Now, there's a seriously kinky girl.

Ms Flynn,

You evidently deserve all the serious humiliation and punishment you receive. Your flagrant display of your vagina and anus warrants it in full. And when your hair was cut off . . . well, that just fully finished your degradation. I shall continue to enjoy your discomfort and the degrading photographs of your vagina and anus at Lupus/RGE.

Keep up your splendid work and keep your knickers down.

Yours

CV, UK

22. FAN MAIL

As you can imagine, spanking models get lots of interesting fan mail and some hate mail too. It ranges from the charming to the obscene. But sometimes I get a message that just makes no sense. Like this one:

From: xx690
Subject: pain

i spank u hard

No name. No punctuation. No information. Is it a promise? A request? How am I supposed to respond to that? More to the point, how did the sender *expect* me to respond? Was he surprised when I didn't? (Or is it sexist of me to assume it was a man?)

Here's another typical one:

is that your bottom in the pic? if so i would like to spank it

Which pic? Where? What if it isn't?

I can understand the motivation behind an abusive message, but ones like that just baffle me.

Once in a while I get a note from someone who clearly doesn't know what to say, but just wants to make contact. These are usually brief, but sincere. And I always try to reply. I'm aware that it takes a lot of courage to approach a celebrity (Me! A celebrity!), even if it's only in writing.

But I'm not sure what to make of this one:

From: Black Stalli
Subject: Spanked in a public place

My girlfriend caught me flirting with two sisters; so she took me into the parking lot of the bar; made me pull down my pant and spanked me with her hair brush right over the back of my motor cycle. It got me so excited.

Well, good for him.

When Adele Haze interviewed me on her blog, she solicited questions from her readers. Here's one from 'Lisa':

I would be interested to hear if Niki is ashamed that everybody can see her naked bottom and even more.

In the unlikely event you were wondering, the answer is no.

This one is sweet, but peculiar:

Your website is fascinating. You are an interesting woman and a beautifully shaped one.

I thanked him for his message and he responded emphatically:

You are very welcome – what I said was true – good luck Dear Lady (you are an UNIGNORABLY shaped woman!)

Thanks. I think.

Here's a Yahoo group post I sincerely enjoyed:

God, you have beautiful feet. I'd love to pamper them, and I'd love to see them caned or whipped. Are there any clips available of this?

Why do I never meet these foot fetishists at events where I'm in agony from wearing five-inch heels all night?

No body part is safe:

I think it would be nice to see your delightful breasts being caned. You are sensation!

They don't all want to abuse me, though:

Just a note to tell you that I too enjoy the glow afterwards. Many a time, I have longed to be right beside you having my bottom reddened as well.

Ah, if only companies would make films where boys and girls get punished together! I'd definitely buy them.

One man wrote to tell me that his local BDSM club liked the Lupus whipping bench so much that they built a replica.

So it looks like I'll be bending over it for a good hard caning. That'll be really special. I'll get to come as close as possible to taking my place alongside you and all the other fabulous Lupus girls.

Not long after that I got an email from someone else who wanted a hard caning. He said:

You girls have given me so much enjoyment I think it only fair to feel firsthand what you go through.

It was the idea of 'fairness' that surprised me. It had never occurred to me to expect that male viewers should know what a severe caning was like. I respect tops who experiment so they know how the implements feel, but surely there was no such obligation when it came to the viewers.

Still, the idea was very erotic. Men wanted to suffer because I had suffered. Because they wanted to know what it was like for me. It's a strange sort of intimacy – connecting with a girl through shared pain.

Many of my favourite emails are from people in other countries. They frequently claim, 'I'm your biggest (Japanese/ Dutch/Russian/etc.) fan.' Even if they're not fluent, they make a valiant effort to speak my language. Their attempts at English can be adorable.

An Italian fan wrote to share his love of being kicked in the balls, comparing it to my enjoyment of the fading pain of a caning. I was sure something had got lost in translation, so I asked him to clarify.

I can't believe you answered me! It's like a dream. Yes, I like to be kicked in the balls, and I think it's like you want to be caned, I think it's the same sensation. Yes, it's very painful, only with a kick a man can fall on the ground for a time, and only a pressure of a female hand squeezing make me full of pain and make me do all what she wants. Have you never kicked a guy in the balls?

About you I really like movies and pictures, and, if you let me say it, I love your body . . . If I make noise to you please don't matter and forgive me.

By now thank you very much to have answered me. I didn't thought it was possible to have contact with people famous like you.

Who could possibly kick such a sweet guy in the balls?

Here's one from a male submissive in Tel Aviv:

Der beautiful Niki.
i see you in film .
i look in your web .
you amazing !!
this is me . . . some photo
i like to be your slave totally .
pleas let me know if we caned meat some day?

I'm always leery when guys attach pictures. You never know if it's going to be a smiling face or a cock shot. I thought the email was charming, but I had no expectations. I downloaded the pics to see an absolutely gorgeous guy with chiselled features and a dancer's physique. In one picture he was kneeling at the feet of a dominatrix. In another he was bound and gagged while she dripped hot wax on his gleaming bare torso. With a slave like that on offer I could easily be tempted!

This came from someone in Greece:

I think it is needless to say that I am one of your thousands of fans, as I think you are getting tonnes of emails every day.

I came across yesterday at your site the photos of your work with pain4fem and I was very happy because they also own a footwhipping site and in my greatest fantasies you would made some footwhipping shootings too . . .

I have no idea why so many men want to see my feet whipped, but I love it.

The majority of my foreign correspondents are German. Most of them speak English fairly well, but they also let me practise my German on them. We'll often have exchanges where each writes in the other's language. Then we correct each other's mistakes. I can only hope they find my fractured German as endearing as I find their fractured English. It's a kooky way to learn a language and as a result my vocabulary is pretty specialised. I don't know how to ask if the train goes to Berlin, but I can certainly beg the headmaster not to cane me!

There's one German man who likes to send me the email equivalent of obscene phone calls. He said he loved to see my shaved '*Muschi*' (I trust that needs no translation) and he asked me repeatedly for pictures of it. I told him he'd have to be satisfied with what he could find online. He gets off on being crude and he especially enjoys describing his favourite pictures to me in graphic detail. (I learned a lot of naughty German slang from him.) I don't think he even knows what I look like, as I'm not in most of the pictures he wants to talk about.

Here's a typical offering:

Was empfindest Du selber dabei, wenn Dich drei Männer breitbeinig festhalten und ein vierter Mann Deine Muschi mit einem Gürtel Spankt . . . und das ziemlich hart . . . so wie es aussieht? Kommt es eigentlich nie vor, dass Dich jemand in so einem Film nicht real fickt . . . gegen Deinen Willen? Bekommst Du oft angebote für Sex?

(What do you feel when three men are holding your legs wide apart and a fourth man spanks your pussy with a belt – quite hard, too, by the look of it? Has it actually never happened before that somebody in such a film has fucked you for real . . . against your will? Do you often get offers for sex?)

I told him that in the first instance he'd confused me with another girl, as usual. I also told him I'd had offers, but they'd never been high enough. I haven't heard from him since.

But the prize for cluelessness has to go to this American, who wrote at 3.30 one afternoon:

From: DonA
Subject: spanking

Hi Niki I'd like to give your bare ass a good caining are you willing? Please let me know. DonA

and then wrote again, two hours later, from a different account:

From: Dandydon
Subject: spanking

Hi Niki, I'd Love to cain your bare ass. Are you willing? please let me know. You can also e-mail me at . . . Hope to hear from you soon. dandydon

I looked at his posts on the spanking forum where he'd written to me. In the space of three months he had started *fourteen* separate threads trawling for play partners. By the last one he'd changed his tune and was looking for a lady to spank *him*. I pictured him blindly sending messages to every female on the forum. A bit like carpet-bombing the job market with résumés in the desperate hope that someone – anyone – will hire you.

Which brings me to . . . Offers! I get an amazing amount of offers for film and photo work. And about 90 per cent of them are pure bullshit. You can usually spot the fantasists and time-wasters at a glance. The guy who went to film school with Spielberg probably isn't for real. Same with the one who wants to fly me first class to Tasmania to shoot the story of a woman sentenced to flogging and transportation in 1837. No script yet, but there are rumours of Tasmanian and Australian Commonwealth funding.

A lot of men just want to enact their fantasy with a girl on camera. You wouldn't believe the number of 'offers' I get along the lines of 'I want to fly you to [insert foreign country] and pay you to let me cane you like they do at Lupus.' Now there's a good plot for a slasher film.

Some unscrupulous men actually film 121s (paid private sessions) without the girl knowing it. (Because if he'd asked, she'd have said no.) In at least one case that I know of, these secret films have turned up on a pay site.

I don't do 121s myself, but that doesn't stop potential customers asking. And I don't mind them asking; I just tell them politely that it's not in my repertoire. One charming man wrote to say he'd lined up several 121s for the next week and he'd love to slot me in there too. How flattering. I said no. His next email assured me that he considered himself 'something of an expert'. I'd have a great time, he insisted, I should give it a chance. Again I said no, this time more firmly. But he kept on. He got pushy, asking what I was afraid of. It was safer than doing a video and he wouldn't hurt me as much. He said I didn't know what I was missing. I had to wonder how often his persistence paid off. Did girls eventually agree out of sheer weariness? My terse response eventually got the message through and he left me alone.

I did consider a 121 once. A gentleman in London wrote to me through one of the spanking forums, hinting at an elaborate fantasy.

I have had a little idea brewing in my mind for several years concerning a particular scene I would like to re-create. It would however require a lady who could take a 'substantial' amount of punishment and pain. From several movies I have seen only Lupus regulars would be sufficient in withstanding this sort of punishment. And, to my knowledge, you are the only English girl who has ever been able to travel and engage in a Lupus production. Maybe you know of some others I could try contacting?

Obviously the girl chosen would be heavily rewarded both for her time and for any work she would lose while she waited for the bruising to subside. I was thinking in the region of £3,000–£3,500 plus any expenses, travel and so on. The entire process should take no longer than a day. 7–8 hours of work. As the amount indicates this is something I greatly wish to pursue – and would even be willing to go higher if necessary. Money is no real obstacle to making this as perfect as I imagine. Even if this entailed hiring two girls for their mutual comfort in such a surrounding.

A seven- to eight-hour roleplay? He'd got my attention. The amount was nothing to sniff at either if he was serious. He seemed sincere and asking if I knew of other girls he could contact lent the whole approach a ring of truth. He was obviously intelligent and educated, which also made it seem genuine.

'Well, I don't do private sessions,' I replied. 'But you've made me curious. I'd love to hear about this fantasy of yours.'

He replied with some personal information by way of introduction. Plausible career, divorced, grown children. He told me of his lifelong fascination with spanking. He said he'd explored the local BDSM scene, but didn't feel at ease with the people there.

The participant would need to be a fairly good actress – as you are – and be able to roleplay for a significant amount of time. I see myself in the role of a student who has been called to a headmistress's office to be disciplined for a misdemeanor. She is a very dominant woman and is dressed in a very prudish way. To the outside eye at least. Under her formal attire though she would be in a corset and suspenders, with sheer black stockings. When I get to her office she lays down what she will do to teach me a lesson. She gloats as she details how she will hurt me.

However I then reveal to her that I have certain 'information' which allows me to reverse the situation and leads to the strict headmistress having to lift her skirt and take a spanking herself. I would delight in my newfound control over her and make my new 'pet' strip and display herself for me – slowly but surely subjecting her to hours of torturous spanking and caning. She would be a strong woman who would do everything she could to remain calm – but the punishments would be to the level where eventually she would be unable to stop herself weeping. And I would delight in breaking her spirit as she had done to so many of my fellow pupils. Her perfect skin would be blistered and bruised and I would take photographs of it happening to keep her in line in the future. She would have her arse cheeks spread and she would be humiliated for my camera knowing that if word of this ever got out she would be publicly humiliated in front of all the pupils – and those pictures would quickly find their way into the wrong hands.

My fantasy is quite strong. I would have to be able to punish until I was satisfied that no matter how hard she tried – she could not do anything but break down and cry by the end. And I would also be keeping a pictorial record of her arse at every stage of the process. From perfect – to battered and bruised.

Wow.

It wasn't really my kind of scene, but what appealed to me was the psychology behind it. It sounded like something that had sprung from an incident in his past. The meticulous detail about how the headmistress was dressed convinced me that this was indeed something he'd been thinking about for a very long time.

Cameron agreed it didn't sound like a wind-up. The tables-turned element was beyond my usual humiliation comfort zone, but I was sure I'd be able to separate myself from the character when it was over. And if I had a friend with me, she could certainly help talk me down if I found it distressing.

I replied, asking if we could meet for lunch to discuss possibilities. He never wrote back. Perhaps simply telling me about it was enough.

As frustrating and annoying as some exchanges can be, they're still harmless. But there's another category altogether: stalkers.

Now, anyone can catch the eye of a jealous, unbalanced obsessive, but women in the sex industry are frequent targets. Strippers often have customers who get just a little too attached, a little too possessive. I discovered the online spanking community during my time as a dancer. I shared my CP fantasies with anyone who would listen, so I often got kinky email from customers and cyber-friends.

One morning when I was home alone I got an email with the subject line 'You're bad'. I assumed it was from one of my new spanko friends. The message said, 'This is what happens to bad people.' I had a slow modem connection in those days and I waited impatiently for the attached image to download, unfurling from top to bottom. 'Bad people' struck me as odd and I was unsettled as the grainy black and white photograph began to reveal itself. It looked like it was taken in an operating theatre and for a moment I wondered if the sender had simply attached the wrong image. I was used to getting spanking pictures, but this wasn't promising.

Finally, my system downloaded enough of the picture for me to see what it was. It wasn't an operating theatre at all; it was an autopsy room. The title of the picture was 'Chew Toy'.

I deleted the horrific image and checked all the doors and windows in a panic. I was terrified to leave the house and terrified to stay. This was someone's idea of fun. I went online and sought refuge in a chat room, where I pleaded with familiar screen names to reassure me that one of them had sent it in a moment of forgivable bad taste. A clueless acquaintance was easier to cope with than the idea of someone trying to freak me out. Of course, none of them had sent it.

I expected more of the same as I became known in the spanking scene, especially once I started doing movies. A couple of weeks before the *Crime and Punishment* shoot, Cameron got a disturbing email at his work account. All it said was 'interesting', but the threat was implicit in the attached URLs: a link to the Lupus site and a link to another website with my real name.

We had no idea who it could be. Clearly someone had been following *my* movements, but the threat was to Cameron. Was it a jealous viewer? How had they tracked us down? Was it someone who knew us personally? Were we about to get a demand from a blackmailer? We had no idea what to do.

Lupus had actually written the role of the American photographer-gangster in *Crime and Punishment* for Cameron, who was excited about being in a film. But in light of the threatening email, in the end we decided that it was just too risky. Cameron traced the email to Washington DC, but the trail went dead there. Whoever it was must have used a library or other public place to send it.

You can't live your life in fear, however, and, once the initial shock wore off, we put the experience behind us and moved on.

Two years later, it was my turn again. This one used a German Hotmail address and signed himself 'Klaus Schmidt'. He said some unpleasant things about Cameron and made it clear he wanted him out of the picture, casually mentioning part of my home address to imply, 'I know where you live.'

Things like this can really mess with your head. They make you doubt your closest friends and they make you paranoid for weeks. The email proved untraceable.

I did my best not to be upset over it. I wanted to believe I'd simply misunderstood the intent. Perhaps Herr Schmidt was an ex-Stasi officer, a man with access to information and the means of finding out anything about a person. Since I'm so open about my edgy fantasies, he might have thought this would be right in my zone.

But I can't fool myself. I know it for what it was: a threat. And there's nothing erotic about that. It's a perfect illustration of the gulf between fantasy and reality.

(journal entry, age 25)

I had a terrible dream last night. It was my dad's birthday and I was going to bake a cake for him. I'd forgotten to get a present or a card, so I went to buy a card at the last minute and the one I got had all these crude and explicit sexual jokes. I thought it was funny, but when I gave it to him he was really embarrassed. He said he'd read it later, trying to hide his discomfort. I was overwhelmed with guilt as I realised how crude it was, so I took it back to the store. I'd completely forgotten about baking a cake.

When I got to the store, a skinny sharp-faced man barred my way. He said he recognised me, knew who I was. I was afraid, but I tried to act calm. I said in this odd stilted voice, 'I'm not the person you've mistaken me for.' But he knew I was lying and he started screaming obscenities at me. All the people in the store were watching and looking at me with disgust. Pointing at me. I had my stun gun with me and I told him I'd use it if he didn't leave me alone. He kept taunting me: 'Do it, tough girl! Do it!' But I was too afraid to do anything because I knew all the people were on his side.

23. WHAT WORKED AND WHAT DIDN'T

W hen I was about six, I was out shopping with my mother. I did something I wasn't supposed to do (damned if I can remember what) and she said, 'If you do that again I'm going to give you the worst spanking of your life.'

I was intrigued by the challenge, burning with curiosity. It was a big red flashing button labelled DO NOT PUSH. But I was at the age where kids start testing boundaries and I had to see if she'd make good on the threat.

I did it again.

She grabbed me by the arm and dragged me in the direction of the restroom. Instantly I regretted my recklessness. Tears welled in my eyes, but I was too frightened to plead. When we got to the restroom, she gripped my arm tightly and raised her right hand up behind me. I held my breath and was surprised when she only gave me a few half-hearted swats over my shorts. It didn't even hurt. I stared at her, baffled. Then I said with all the innocent frankness of a child, 'That wasn't the worst spanking of my life.'

I wasn't being cheeky; it was merely an interested observation. She couldn't do anything but laugh.

Then there was the time I wandered too far down the street. I was nine or ten. My parents were overprotective and I had no idea I wasn't supposed to go 'all the way down there'. I followed whatever butterfly I was chasing until I heard my father calling me to come inside. My sister and I had been playing outside with Brad and Kristy, the kids who lived across the street. They all watched me, wide-eyed, as I followed my dad into the house, sick with worry. I was afraid, but, when I got inside, all he did was tell me not to go that far again. I remember thinking, *That's all?* though I didn't say it. Disoriented, I promised to stay close to the house. Then I went back outside to join the others.

Brad and Kristy instantly demanded to hear the details of the punishment.

'Nothing happened,' I said, still surprised nothing had.

Kristy narrowed her eyes at me. 'You're lying.'

'I'm not! I swear I'm not!'

'We always tell you when we get the belt,' she said, pouting.

'I'd tell you if there was anything to tell,' I insisted. 'Look, I haven't even been crying.'

I couldn't convince her, though. And in later years I wondered if her obsession with hearing the details meant she was One Of Us.

I wasn't abused, but my memories of actual childhood punishments aren't pleasant. I truly believe my parents only did what they thought was best. They were both of the 'never did me any harm' school of thought. I like to think they were simply misguided.

My mother and I had a stormy relationship. She wasn't very good at controlling her temper and she often punished in anger. She kept score too. Punishment didn't necessarily mean I was forgiven. The past could be dredged up again in any argument.

By contrast, most spanking roleplay is caring and it's never angry or out of control. There is always closure at the end; hugs are standard after a scene. It's an idealised version of 'how it should be done', though most kinky people feel spanking is appropriate only for consenting adults.

Once when I was fifteen I was feeling desperately lonely for a boyfriend. (I'd never had one.) My mother was going to drop Jessie and me off at the movies, so I decided to dress up for a change. I put on a vintage black flapper dress with tons of fringe. Then I added black stockings and the low heels I'd worn to a school dance. I even put on lipstick, which I hated. Posing in the mirror, I thought I looked older, sophisticated.

'You are *not* going out looking like a streetwalker!' was my mother's reaction.

I was truly taken aback. I fled to my room in tears, my confidence annihilated. We did not go to the movies.

Mother/daughter scenes are a hard limit for me. I won't play them and I can't even watch them. It's a dynamic I simply can't eroticise. However, father/daughter scenes are fine. My father was harmless. He only ever disciplined me a handful of times and it hurt him more than me. I made sure of that.

Hand-spankings were tolerable, but the belt hurt. Jessie and I would scream at the top of our lungs whenever we were punished. We wanted the neighbours to hear and call the police. We also believed that 'sound drowns out pain'. It's actually kind of funny to think back on it because, now that I have some perspective, it really wasn't all that hard.

Our melodramatic cries didn't faze my mother, but they upset my father something rotten. In later years my mom told me that he was in tears after one particular performance of mine. It was the last time he ever punished me physically. If I'd known at the time, I'd have considered it a glorious personal victory.

OK, confession time. I've said I was Goody Two Shoes in school and for the most part I was. I never tried drugs or skipped school. I was never rude to teachers. I never fought. I never messed around with boys. I usually did my homework. But I did have two serious vices. I was a shoplifter and a pathological liar.

Shoplifting was like my rape fantasies; it gave me an erotic rush. A shrink would have called it kleptomania and said that I secretly wanted to be caught and punished. Maybe he'd have been right.

It was a phase I eventually grew out of and I count myself lucky I was never caught. It's a potent fantasy for me now. I remember vividly the cold sweat and pounding heart that went along with every meaningless item I slipped into my pockets or let fall into my purse. The high when I got away with it. It translates as sexual excitement when I think back on it. I remember the fear of a heavy hand clapping down on my shoulder. The deep voice of the policeman telling me I need to accompany him to the station. The knowledge that I've really done it this time . . . It's powerful stuff.

Shoplifting was a cheap physical thrill. But lying was more complex; it was all about fantasy. Or more precisely, escaping reality. I simply liked telling stories. On camping trips I was the one who could be counted on to tell ghost stories that would keep the other girls up all night in terror. I adored scaring them. Soon I was casting myself in the stories, describing the cold spot in our house where someone had once been murdered or the voice you could hear coming out of the drainpipe. Firsthand accounts always carry more weight than urban legends about men with hooks for hands.

My parents had taken me house-hunting with them once and I was thrilled to discover a cobwebbed attic with a trapdoor. My imagination ran amok and I wove an elaborate story about a box of dusty old books I'd found up there. One book had a page with its corner turned down, so I flipped it open to be confronted by the illustration of a giant rat. The picture was monochrome, but the eyes had been coloured a lurid red – with blood, I was sure. I stared at it, mesmerised. Then I saw the creature blink. As I told this chilling tale to my rat-phobic audience, I produced a book I'd been hiding under my pillow. I opened it to the dogeared page and sure enough, there was the very same red-eyed rat.

'And if you look really closely,' I said in a whisper, urging the other girls to lean in. 'You can see it – BLINK!' Here I snapped the book shut with a loud pop and my audience shrieked in terror. It wasn't exactly Ramsey Campbell, but it was enough to scare a gaggle of nine-year-olds. And they always came back for more.

It started innocently enough, but I soon began to depend on lies as a way of making myself interesting. Most importantly though, lying taught me how to escape punishment. Occasionally I'd get caught, but it was always better to try to lie my way out of it first. The trouble was, I wasn't very good at it.

For some reason, my parents never spanked me for lying. I don't know why. They had a different punishment for that, although they never imposed it on my sister. They made me write lines.

'I will not lie' is hardly the worst sentence to have to write, but 500 is a big number. I remember spending whole Saturdays in my room, scribbling those four little words ever more illegibly as the numbers bled into one another and the words began to lose their meaning.

Or did they?

Training is repetition and so is programming. Brainwashing. No amount of physical pain ever made the slightest difference to me. It hurt at the time and it put me on my guard for the next couple of weeks. I certainly did my best not to get caught again. But it never radically altered my behaviour the way those interminable lines did. By the time I graduated from high school,

I was virtually incapable of telling a lie. The very thought was so abhorrent that even a harmless 'white lie' would make me feel physically ill. There's some sound psychology in *A Clockwork Orange*.

Over time I did learn to lie again, especially when I had to pretend to like vanilla sex and have porn-star orgasms. But it was extremely stressful for me. If I told someone a lie, I'd be consumed with guilt as well as paranoia that I wouldn't remember it later. I just couldn't cope with the anxiety and the only solution was to stop lying.

Unfortunately, there are situations where it's necessary. Like online interviews where you don't want to resurrect the past. And all subsequent interviews where you have to maintain the fiction you've created. I still hate having to lie and sometimes I feel that insidious conditioning struggling to turn the anxiety into nausea. But I've learned to resist it.

I was cured, all right.

Dear Niki,

Be courageous! If somebody want to say that you are a torturer of poor Czech girls, he must be very stupid. And don't be afraid because you are very popular in Czech Republic and it's honour for us that you are working here. You are our darling!

Kisses,

Robert, Czech Republic

24. I HAVE NOTHING TO WEAR

Choosing what to pack for a shoot can be a daunting task. I never know what I'm going to need and I've learned not to rely on the companies to provide wardrobe. Lupus is the exception.

Cameron and I have quite a collection of costumes and uniforms – school and military. Just to give you an idea – I have five crisp white shirts, three different school ties, sixteen pleated skirts and kilts in various colours and styles, two Japanese school uniforms, one Taiwanese uniform and one pair of short trousers and a schoolboy cap for when I'm feeling boyish. The military uniforms and headmaster's gown take up even more space. We had to build a walk-in wardrobe to accommodate all this. There's another wardrobe in the bedroom and two large chests of drawers filled with clothes – mostly mine.

My underwear collection is even more impressive. I was going to make an estimate, but decided I'd do an inventory rather than risk inflating the numbers. Are you ready?

School knickers: 12 pairs. A proper school number, that. I can see the regulations now.

Thongs: 23. That's a hell of a lot for a girl who doesn't wear thongs.

Dance thongs: 6. These are ones I used to dance in at the club and just couldn't part with. It would have been more, but my favourite two were stolen from a laundromat in New York. I hope they gave the wanker some pleasure.

Everything else (panties, boyshorts and French knickers): 73. Well, 76 if you count the Victorian split-crotch pantalets, frilly bloomers and latex hot pants.

Disposable: 15. These are old pairs I keep for scenes where my panties are cut or ripped from me.

About a third of this stuff has never even been worn. And as I write this there's another shipment of 10 on the way from Victoria's Secret. Hey, there are worse addictions. More expensive ones too.

My shoe collection, while ample, can't compete (36 pairs at the last count).

If I'm going to be doing lots of clips, I need to take a variety of different outfits. Here's the inventory of my suitcase for a typical shoot:

School uniform. English style: white shirt, striped blue tie, navy blue pleated skirt, white socks and black shoes. Four pairs of school knickers. (Can't be too careful; *nothing* displays wetness and arousal like white cotton!)

An elegant dress or two in the unlikely event I get to play a grownup.

Teen slutwear – a selection of sexy tops, skirts and shorts.

Jeans. Ultra-tight jeans. Always.

Pyjamas. Cutesy ones for the shoot and practical ones to sleep in.

Cheerleader uniform. I always take it, but I've never worn it.

Underwear. 15 to 20 pairs of sexy knickers and a couple of thongs. Not that I'll wear them all; I just like having loads to choose from.

Shoes – school shoes, heels, ballet slippers and running shoes.

Oversize men's German army shirt for cover-up between nude scenes.

Any personal implements or props I want to use.

Palmer's Cocoa Butter lotion for moisturising before and after every scene.

Dermablend makeup in several shades – absolutely the best for covering tattoos, bruises and blemishes.

Arnica gel for any bruising after the shoot.

Aloe vera for cuts and abrasions.

First aid kit. (Strange we may be, but always responsible.)
Comfy baggy trousers to go home in.

But even with all my careful planning and packing, chances are I'm just going to wind up naked anyway.

Dear Mom and Dad,

I love England. Everyone here is really nice.

Today I shot for a company called Firm Hand. Samantha Woodley and I played bratty American girls sent to a strict English school. Boy, is my bottom sore! But it was lots of fun. I had to change my knickers twice because the wet patch would have been obvious on film.

I'm sure you'd agree that our characters deserved everything we got! I mean, I'd never have got away with behaving like that when I was a kid. Remember? But it's cool now because this time I'm a grownup. This time I actually *want* it. The funny thing is, some people think it's sick. That's what really confuses me. It's sick if it's done to consenting adults who find it hot, but not when it's done to non-consenting children? Weird.

Anyway, I'm having a lovely time. Wish you were here.

Your loving daughter

*   *   *

Dear Mom and Dad,

England is wonderful, and I have a new job. You know all those coffee-table books with artsy nude photos? Well, it's a bit like that.

Don't worry, it's nothing pornographic. The photographers are very professional, and it pays pretty well too. Who knows? You might even see me on the Net!

*   *   *

Dear Mom and Dad,

I'm a spanking model. There. I said it. Do you hate me now?

*   *   *

Dear Mom and Dad,

I've got something to tell you. I'm dying. (Actually, I'm not really dying. I'm just a porn star. But look at in context.)

*   *   *

Dear PostSecret,

I wish I could tell my parents I'm famous.

25. A DEAD BEE MAKES NO HONEY

A dele Haze is crying in the bunk below me. She's just been admitted to the prison and put into my cell.

Intakes are a painful process. The screws are all sadistic power trippers, especially the evil Matron. I'd been admitted the day before and I really set Matron off. Sentenced to thirteen years for arson, I haven't spoken since my arrest. The jury didn't buy the insanity plea, so I wound up in here. Matron and Officer Kennedy tried to get me to speak at my intake, but I only clung to Horatio in stubborn silence as they thrashed me.

I feel sorry for the convicted murderess below me, so I slip into her bed to offer Horatio to her for comfort. They'd let me keep the teddy bear because they thought it might keep me out of trouble.

Adele sniffles and gives me a grateful smile.

'What's your name?' she asks.

When I don't answer she assumes I don't speak English.

'*Parles-tu français?*'

I'm in my own world, though, affectionately stroking my cellmate's leg. One gets so lonely in prison, you see.

Adele tries a variety of languages until she hits on Russian. The exotic music affects me and I sigh, my body responding to the lyrical tones. I can't understand a word as she murmurs liquidly to me, but it doesn't matter. Her hands are telling me all I need to know.

Adele draws her fingers down my leg, slipping my sock off. She kisses my foot gently before closing her lips around my toes, sucking them one by one, pressing her warm tongue into the soft webbing between them. I arch into the sensation, gripping the springs of the bunk above me. With her tongue she traces a path up the delicate skin of my sole. I throw my head back as she sends sparks through my foot and up the length of my leg. Inflamed, I take over.

I push her onto her back and lie on top of her, kissing her hungrily. Twisting a hand in her long dark hair, I expose her pale throat. Adele moans and writhes beneath me as she feels my teeth. I pin her wrists down and grind against her. She unzips my red prison tunic, stripping it off and caressing the warm flesh she's exposed as she presses her knee up between my—

'Right, I think enough's enough here.'

Officer Lewis. This is the most hated man on the Net.

Bars and Stripes is the brainchild of ex-ballet dancer Leia-Ann Woods. Her partner in crime is a charming guy named Michael Stamp. Together they created a prison website with recurring characters and a serialised storyline. It's the nearest thing there is to a spanking soap opera. Leia is the prison's top dog, 'Mrs Woods', and Michael is the voyeuristic prison governor, known only as Number One.

Adele and I had worked together for Northern Spanking Institute one chilly winter weekend and it was the most fun I'd ever had on a shoot. It was like a weekend of non-stop roleplay for both of us. I played a cat burglar and a ballerina. I got to do a pole-dance. I even topped Adele in two schoolgirl scenes.

Northern Spanking is run by Lucy McLean, a lively Glaswegian blonde with a terrific sense of fun. Paul Kennedy is Lucy's husband and business partner. They've been in the scene all their adult lives and they're true aficionados. Lucy has a real passion for filmmaking and recently went to film school to hone her skills. Paul is a stills photographer. Together they make a perfect team.

It's always a joy to shoot with companies that work to raise the genre above the level of mere porn. Don't get me wrong; porn is great and if all you want to see is a bottom being smacked, there's plenty of material around. But for a lot of us, CP is nothing without the context. At the shoot Lucy gave Adele and me free rein in writing our own stories and scenarios. All her girls are for real. No vanilla models allowed.

Adele and I met Michael at the shoot and he showed us some episodes from Bars and Stripes. The two companies share everything – tops, bottoms, locations and camera crew. Lucy plays the sadistic Matron on B&S while Paul plays the senior guard.

The soap opera format of B&S involves the viewers in an interactive fantasy. People who join the website are greeted as members of the prison Board of Governors and they can follow links to the cellblock, the sickbay or the intake office. They can read the inmates' rap sheets and make suggestions for how offenders should be dealt with. They can even read Mrs Woods's secret prison diary.

'Number One' often gets emails from viewers warning him about which girls are selling drugs or who's planning a breakout. One gentleman insisted that sweet submissive Rhiannon Diablo be broken straight away by twenty strokes of the birch. 'She's one of those "butter wouldn't melt in her mouth" types,' he wrote. 'But she'll cause more trouble than half the tougher inmates together.'

Another man kindly offered to take Gina Moon's punishment for her; he thought she was innocent. And another had a replica B&S prison tunic made for his wife and sent Michael a photo.

Best of all are the reports he gets about Matron. 'Why can't you see what she's doing to those poor girls?' one viewer asked, incredulous. 'You need to keep an eye on her!' Lucy often has to reassure people that she's not really evil, that Matron is just a character she plays.

Adele and I fell in love with the concept. We were instantly hooked. 'How do we get sent to this prison?' we demanded to know.

'Easy,' Michael told us. 'Choose your crimes and we'll book you.'

I'm an unabashed fan of the women-in-prison (WiP) exploitation films of the 70s. There's invariably a resident psycho in the cast and that was who I wanted to play. I thought it would be fun if I didn't speak for several episodes. Then Matron could do something to trigger a psychotic break and I would explode. I decided that carrying a teddy bear would be a nice touch and it would give me the perfect thing to come undone over. (I confess I stole the idea from the WiP classic *Reform School Girls*, though Leia's a much sexier queen bee than Wendy O Williams.)

Adele wanted to be a murderess. Taking *Basic Instinct* as her inspiration, she made herself an eccentric horror novelist who'd allegedly chopped her old headmaster into tiny bits. The same thing had happened to a character in one of her books, so the police were suspicious.

I was a little shy about doing a love scene with another girl. Despite my early sexual experience, I'm not bi. This time it wouldn't just be moans in the dark, like in my scene with Bailey. This time there would be actual kissing and caressing. But Adele and I were good friends and we were up for the adventure. You can't have women in prison without the girlie stuff; it's like a Bond film without the gadgets. We spent a lot of time discussing what we should do. I knew what would work for me; I just couldn't be sure it would work for her.

Oh, the footsie stuff was no problem. She was happy to do that. But I needed something to incite me to passion in the first place.

'What would turn you on?' she asked.

'Um, well, I . . .'

'Tell me.'

'Well, you know how I have this thing about foreign languages, right?'

'Mm-hmm.'

'Maybe if you . . . you know . . . said stuff in Russian or something . . .'

A huge grin spread across her face. 'I think I could manage that.'

We joked with everyone the night before about needing lots and lots of rehearsal time, but the truth was that we did. We were both so nervous about it. Our first love scene! It had to be well choreographed or we'd just be knocking our foreheads together clumsily, stammering and giggling. Viewers have no idea how much planning and preparation can go into these scenes.

Our elaborate storyline extended far beyond what we'd be able to shoot. We'd decided that I would develop an obsessive fixation on my cellmate, stalking her and sending her weird notes. Adele would find other 'special friends' in prison, making me jealous and dangerous. In dripping red paint I scrawled A DEAD BEE MAKES NO HONEY on a scrap of newspaper (a nod to my favourite WiP film, *The Big Doll House*), intending to send it to Adele as a threat.

We did a quick walk-through before shooting so that Michael and Leia could arrange the cameras. Stephen Lewis was charmed by our devotion to duty. He breaks up all the prison lesbian scenes; hence his reputation as the most hated man in the business. But it provides a perfect excuse for a CP scene and that's ultimately what B&S viewers are there to see.

'How long should I let them go on before I bust it up?' Lewis asked.

'Oh, ten minutes should do it,' Michael said.

Adele and I gaped at each other. 'Ten minutes?'

'Michael, that's an eternity!' Leia said, laughing. 'Not that I'd mind.' (Mrs Woods likes her 'private moments' with fellow inmates. All part of showing them who's boss.)

'OK, OK, maybe five or six minutes, then.'

That sounded manageable.

'Action!'

Crying. Teddy bear. Russian dialogue. Kissing. Foot stuff. It was all going well, just as we'd rehearsed it. I pinned my cellmate down, kissing her ardently while she moaned beneath me. Though her mouth was occupied, I was still hearing Russian in my head. And responding.

I unzipped her tunic enough to expose her black lace bra, drawing my fingers lightly down her face, her throat, her chest.

Gasp, sigh. More Russian. Pant, pant.

She peeled me out of my tunic and I was just about to take hers off as well when Lewis interrupted us. I was genuinely startled; I didn't realise he was right behind us. He'd been standing there watching our little show for ages.

'Nice work, ladies,' Leia said.

Adele said she'd had to pretend she couldn't see him, but I'd been completely oblivious. Ah, the magic of foreign tongues.

'Hey, you want to know how long that was?' Michael asked. 'Ten minutes exactly!'

Adele and I looked at each other sheepishly.

'Yeah, well,' we mumbled. 'Acting, you know . . .'

The next day we were sent with Leia to clean one of the guards' offices with toothbrushes. And when I saw Adele flirting with Leia, I flew into a jealous rage. She was *my* special friend! Leia and I went at it with fur flying while Adele tried to get between us. The screws arrived to break it up and Lewis dragged Leia off to solitary.

Adele and I were shaking all over. Wired. We felt like we'd been given a shot of adrenalin straight to the heart.

'Yeah, fight scenes do that,' Lucy said knowingly. 'It was only about two minutes, but I'll bet it felt like forever!'

It had.

Matron and Kennedy tore a strip off Adele and me, taking it in turns to show us that they wouldn't tolerate a prison riot. They thrashed us both, using everyone's favourite B&S implement, the Strap of Joy. It's a ferocious-looking rough leather strap that makes plenty of noise, but doesn't actually hurt all that much. It's good to have an implement the tops can wield full-force without damage, especially on bottoms that have suffered several punishments already.

But the cane came next, and there is no Cane of Joy. The murderess and the arsonist howled and sobbed as the rattan bit into their tender cheeks again and again. This was an iffy scene because of the handcuffs. The BBFC has funny ideas about 'association of sex with non-consensual restraint'. But who said anything about sex? Adele and I were adamant; no stuffy censor was going to deprive us of our prison abuse fantasy!

Through it all Horatio lay helpless on the desk, a silent witness to our suffering. Suddenly Matron got an evil look in her eye.

'You want your bear?' she asked sweetly.

I pleaded with my eyes as she held him just out of my reach. Then she tore him limb from limb.

It looks simple on film, but there was far more to it than that. I had scoured the local charity shops for the perfect bear and Horatio had a jointed neck and legs. I thought that would make the destruction easier. But modern children's toys are engineered like battleships. We played tug-o'-war with him the night before to loosen the joints, but the tempered steel wouldn't budge. In the end Michael had to take a hacksaw to the poor creature, dismembering him and leaving it to Lucy to stitch him back together. The fragile Franken-Bear had to be handled very carefully until the crucial scene or he'd fall apart.

Horatio's dismemberment broke my silence and what was left of my sanity. I was sent to Matron for shock treatment and when she left me unattended for a moment, I ripped open the feather pillow in her sickbay. I hadn't anticipated such a mess. The thing literally exploded. I tried lamely to scoop the feathers back into the pillowcase, but it was too late.

'You little maniac!' Matron shrieked. 'This is prison property!'

She made me kneel on the bed in the drift of feathers while she vowed to give me the thrashing of my life. Every time I kicked I sent feathers swirling into the air. At one particularly hard stroke

I lurched forwards and got a face full of them. They were everywhere – in my hair, in my underwear and all over the bed and floor. Last I heard, they were still finding feathers on the set.

No one has ever complained about *my* treatment, but plenty of people were concerned about the treatment of the bear.

Section 6: Good Character Requirement

Have you ever been charged or indicted with a criminal offence?

Have you ever been involved in the commission, preparation or organisation of war crimes, crimes against humanity or genocide?

Have you ever been involved in financing, planning, preparation, commission or attempted commission of terrorist acts or in supporting acts of terrorism?

Have you engaged in any other activities which might be relevant to the question of whether you are a person of good character?

Application for UK Residence Permit

26. PARANOIA

'Am I a person of good character?' I asked Cameron.

'What, by Victorian standards?'

'No. By the standards of the UK Immigration and Nationality Directorate.'

We stared at the archaic wording, at a loss. We couldn't find any definition of 'good character' on the Home Office website. How were we supposed to know what the British government considered good character? I wasn't about to post the question on the spanking forums. After careful consideration, we agreed that being spanked on camera did not put me in the same category as people guilty of war crimes, genocide and terrorism. (We did find a definition eventually; it's mostly about obeying laws and paying taxes.)

When SOL imported Lauren, Venus and Darling for their Great American Girl Project, one of my stipulations was that they maintain the fiction that I'd flown in with them. In reality, I simply drove down to Yorkshire from my home up north. Oh, I wasn't in the country illegally. But I wanted to keep a low profile so the Home Office would have no reason to deny my residence permit. I'd jumped through all their hoops and paid their extortionate fees, but Cameron suggested that it was safer not to say where I really lived. I'd already claimed on the forums that I lived in Prague. That was to keep my real location secret – mainly from stalkers.

It became an elaborate game of misinformation. I'd been living in the UK long enough to adopt British spelling and idioms, but in my posts and Lupus articles I'd made a conscious effort to revert to American spelling. When people asked where I lived, I said, 'Oh, I bounce around a lot. Prague. New York. London.' In the Pierson interview I'd said that the idea for *Exchange Student* sprang from having been an exchange student in London. That explained why I spent so much time in the UK.

I hated not being able to share the simplest detail – where I lived – with my fellow spankos. When Cameron and I went to London for parties and events we occasionally took trusted people into our confidence. And a lot of my Czech and German friends knew. They were unlikely to have any dealings with the Home Office.

The question haunted me. Good character. Who was to judge? The idea that I could be denied residence on the basis of an alternative lifestyle was deeply offensive. But it wasn't just my visa that was at stake. Cameron's employer wouldn't be happy to discover that his girlfriend was – well, a porn star. Neither of us worked with children or government secrets, but it was still a concern, still a reason to be paranoid.

I almost got deported once, shortly after I'd arrived in England and well before I became a spanking model. Cameron and I had flown to Amsterdam overnight to see a friend of his and when we got back the next day, the bookish little man who checked my passport decided to give me a hard time. He badgered me with questions for nearly an hour before issuing me a slip of paper. It said I was a person 'liable to be detained' and that I had not officially been admitted to the UK. I had to report the following day for further interrogation.

On paper it sounds like the plot of a CP film (Please, sir, I'll do *anything* to stay in the country!), but it was about as erotic as a job interview. The immigration officers – there were two of them – seemed convinced I was working in the UK (I wasn't) and they hounded me about my relationship with Cameron. At the time we we weren't really sure ourselves where our relationship was going, and we certainly didn't want to share it with immigration officers. But my questioners thought that was suspicious.

'He flew you over here and to Amsterdam? And you're staying in his house rent-free? That's very generous of him. Are you with him for the money?'

I couldn't believe the things they were asking and insinuating. I hadn't even made my first film yet, so I had nothing to hide. But situations like that are designed to make you feel like a criminal.

In the end I convinced them that I wasn't working or sponging off the welfare system and they released me. As interrogations go, it was pretty lame; they missed a lot of tricks. There were no uniforms, no peaked caps, no light to shine in my eyes. And even though there were two of them, they didn't play the good cop/bad cop game. Amateurs.

However, once I started making CP movies, the prospect of another 'interview' terrified me. I'd been a good girl most of my life, so my new underground lifestyle was difficult to reconcile with my everyday existence. I felt like a fugitive every time I went to the airport, in hats and dark glasses in case my alter ego's picture was tacked up behind the check-in desk. I dreaded the immigration queue at both ends, where I might be asked 'the purpose of my visit' to Prague. My *frequent* visits to Prague.

And there was the ever-present shadow of my parents. The most innocent question could send me into a panic.

'So, what did you do last weekend?'

'Oh, just hung around the house, really. Did some gardening. Watched a couple of movies.' Our vanilla friends must think we're the most boring couple on the planet.

Of course I have a life outside the kink, but my daily routine revolves around my alternative career. My website, blog and Yahoo group consume a lot of my time and email can sometimes take days to get on top of. There are offers of work to consider and schedules to coordinate, not to mention personal correspondence with friends, both kinky and vanilla. I have two email accounts to juggle. I'm always afraid of slipping up – signing 'love, Niki' on an email to my dad or accidentally attaching the wrong set of holiday snaps. Managing my identities is a full-time job.

Having vanilla visitors means sanitising the house and making sure we haven't left toys or bondage equipment lying around. Or spanking porn. We have to block access to the walk-in wardrobe and 'kink cupboard' and take down any naughty fridge poetry composed by kinky visitors. As for my computer . . . The only solution is not to allow anyone near it who doesn't know what we're into.

Worst of all are vanilla social gatherings. All those innocuous questions that normal people can answer without breaking into a cold sweat.

'So how did you two meet?'

On three separate occasions I'd just taken a bite of food when this was asked. I made a big show of chewing and indicating that I couldn't possibly be so rude as to talk with my mouth full. Cameron's better at handling that one.

'It was in an antique shop in New York,' he said coolly every time. And promptly changed the subject. We *could* say we met on the Net, but that would raise eyebrows. And people would ask where. A historical re-enactment society's website?

The 'where we met' question was always tricky because before we came up with the antique shop we'd simply cited 'mutual friends'. But that opened the door to even more questions. Who? Where? When?

'Can't we just say we met in rehab?' I'd lamented once. 'That's bound to make them wish they'd never asked.'

One time I got cornered at a party and my chatty companion asked where we'd met. I blanched and looked wildly around for Cameron, who was nowhere in sight. 'Ah,' I said, taking a big gulp of my vodka tonic, trying to remember my lines. 'It was in New York.'

'Really? When was that?'

Another gulp. Rattle of ice. *Please offer to get me another drink before I have to answer.* 'Oh, um ... about ...' It was torture! And all the while I was picturing Cameron off in another corner, sweating out the same question under the lights. And afterwards our interrogators would compare notes to see if our stories matched.

I did eventually come out to my mother. Sort of. I took her to lunch and she asked enough little probing questions to show she knew Cameron and I didn't have a conventional relationship. She knew I'd been a dancer and I didn't want her to think we'd met at the club. (My dad still had no idea.)

'Well, all right,' I began reluctantly. 'We didn't really meet in an antique shop.'

'I thought that sounded far-fetched.'

'We met online.'

'What, in a chat room or something?'

'Something like that.'

She obviously wasn't able to guess or she would have. I was stuck. I'd have to offer the information rather than simply confirm her suspicions.

'It's a bit of an alternative lifestyle,' I said.

She didn't respond; she just waited for me to continue. I glanced forlornly at my second empty margarita glass and scanned the room for our waiter.

'You know what S&M is, right?'

Her forehead creased slightly, though she was trying hard to keep a poker face. 'Yes.'

'Well, it's not really whips and chains we're into,' I said, choosing my words carefully. 'It's more . . . domestic.'

'Domestic?' She pondered that and took a sip from her half-empty glass. My throat felt parched.

'Roleplay,' I offered. 'Kind of like I used to do in drama. But kinky. Especially school scenes.'

She nodded. 'I think I understand.'

I smiled with relief.

'Like seducing a teacher?'

My smile wilted. 'Um, no, not quite.' It was just too embarrassing. There was no way I could tell her.

The waiter finally noticed my frantic waving and halfway through my third drink I'd suggested enough clues that she was starting to get the picture. She even said the S-word, but I was too mortified to look her in the eye. I just nodded, my face blazing. I managed to tell her about Shadow Lane in a roundabout way, characterising it as the kinky equivalent of a Star Trek convention.

'It's all safe, sane and consensual,' I reassured her, parroting the creed like a glazed-eyed cult member. 'So you don't have to worry about me.'

To her credit, she didn't seem upset. Uncomfortable, but not traumatised. Looking back, she was probably more afraid than I was. There are plenty of freakier things I could have been into.

Hi Niki. I got *Stalin 2* last week and can only say OMG!!! Incredible. As expected, you were great and so were the other girls. But I hope that is your last Lupus film. What can you do to top that? Actual death is not an option.

LV-Racer, Las Vegas

27. WE'RE ALL MAD HERE

The six of us stand in a line in the dark corridor, huddled close together. We're frightened by the sirens and gunshots outside. The guards have dragged us from our beds and now they stand over us with guns. They wear white lab coats over their uniforms. They're not doctors, but we're under their care in this place. At their mercy.

The noises were terrifying, but the silence is worse. Even the dogs have stopped barking. We don't dare move. Two guards enter, bearing a stretcher between them. They set it down in front of us and we turn away in horror at the blood-soaked body of a girl dressed in the same yellow madhouse pyjamas we wear.

Suddenly a door opens at the far end of the corridor and a shaft of cold light unfurls along the floor. The chief warden marches to where we stand, trembling and tearful. He gazes impassively at the dead girl and his cold gaze sweeps along the line as he looks hard at each of us in turn.

'If you try to escape,' he says, his voice eerily calm, 'you'll end up like her.'

In *Stalin 2* Nikolaja was defiant. She believed that her stubbornness and indignation would ultimately prove her innocence to the Communist interrogators. She was wrong. She had no idea what she was up against. But while it was scary and intense in the moment, it was easy to shake it off afterwards. Once we'd filmed the mock execution it was time for lunch and we were all back to chatting and joking around.

Stalin 3 took me much further. This time Nikolaja was broken. And this time it wasn't so easy to come back.

The story is told in flashbacks as a documentary of Nikolaja's experiences in custody in Czechoslovakia. After sentencing her to death, the government worried that executing a British subject might cast their regime in a poor international light. So they dumped her in a psychiatric hospital. Using archival footage of a filmed statement Nikolaja made after her release through a hostage exchange, the documentary details the cruelty of the guards in the madhouse.

I was amazed at the scope of the project. There were more than twenty characters, including six other female inmates. Five of them would be caned as the film progressed. *Stalin 2* had been the biggest Lupus project to date, but *Stalin 3* was a giant step beyond that. The story had four intersecting timelines, and the most intense scenes Pavel Šťastný had ever written.

The film opens with Nikolaja's arrival at the hospital, where she thinks she will be executed. Instead, she is shoved into a filthy cell with restraints on the iron bunk bed. She falls apart as she realises that the torment isn't over. She has no way of knowing if it will ever end.

The inmates wear identical yellow pyjamas with no elastic in the pants. Ostensibly it's to hamper escape attempts, but really it's just one of the many ways the guards humiliate them. They force the girls to run through the corridors with their hands on their heads, shouting at them when they stop to pull their pants up. Conversation is forbidden and girls who break that rule are sent to the correction room. For caning, of course.

The inmates spend their days sitting around with nothing to do. One day a girl named Libuše is brought into the day room. She smiles at Nikolaja, risking the wrath of the guards. It is the first kindness Nikolaja has known in years. Libuše is in the madhouse because she wanted to become a nun, so the guards take particular delight in abusing her. She is raped and beaten when she resists. Seeing this, Nikolaja doesn't resist when it's her turn. As a result, Libuše feels betrayed and turns away. Shortly afterwards, she kills herself in the shower. Nikolaja feels responsible.

Her fate is changed when the West Germans capture a Czech

spy (Pavel) and agree to a hostage exchange. On an abandoned border crossing, Nikolaja is finally released.

The psychodrama was intimidating enough, but I was terrified to learn that I would be narrating the entire story. It rattled me more than the thought of another Lupus caning. At least my lines were all in English.

Bailey was visiting us when Lupus sent me the script. We'd become good friends since the *Conspiracy* shoot in Denver and she'd come to stay with Cameron and me for a couple of weeks. When the script arrived in my inbox, I printed it out and we all curled up in bed with a bottle of wine to read it, passing it on page by page.

'Wow,' said Bailey. 'Um, wow. Is Lupus always so political?'

Cameron nodded, engrossed in the torments I was going to suffer. 'It's one of their hallmarks.'

It's always slightly unsettling to read a script for a film I'm already cast in. There's something inescapable about it, like reading the sentence for a judicial punishment. It's thrilling to see how completely someone holds my fate in his hands. It feels like there's no backing out.

Over the next few days I read and reread the script, wondering if I could learn all those lines. They weren't sure how much would be voiceover and how much would be me talking to the camera, so I had to memorise it all. I hoped that the narration would be shot last, so I could at least remember the actual events as I talked about them. But when I got the shooting schedule I was dismayed to learn that I would be doing all my narration halfway through the three-day shoot – before experiencing the most traumatic episodes in the story.

It was our second Easter in Prague, two years since my first shoot. I'd come so far so fast. One moment I was just a kinky girl; the next I was a film star.

In retrospect it's weird that it never felt weird. I didn't have sex with them, but I routinely had intimate encounters with strangers. I was often spanked by men or women I'd just met that day. It seemed perfectly natural to me. I guess it's a bit like hard sports. You'd play football with strangers, right? There's close physical contact, but nothing overtly sexual.

I've just never felt that proprietary about my body. Or my partner's. Cameron and I relished each other's accounts of scenes – some sexual, some not – with friends. The one thing we agreed was off limits was unprotected sex.

I'd been sheltered all my life, so it's little wonder I was fascinated by danger. But, true to form, with me it was always *safe* danger. My self-destructive adolescence seemed like someone else's life. Now I was living my dreams. And I had an understanding partner to share every experience with.

The night Cameron and I arrived we met up with several of the Lupus crew for dinner. Zbyšek, Thomas and Pavel wanted to discuss some of the scenes before the next day's shoot. It was always difficult for Zbyšek, directing in two languages, so he wanted a chance to talk to me one-on-one. Perhaps they also wanted to make sure I was of sound enough mind to handle it.

Pavel gave me an Easter gift of five *pomlázky* he'd made himself. The waiter grinned hugely at the sight: a girl clutching five braided switches, sitting at a table surrounded by five men. Truly a lamb amongst wolves.

'This is the darkest story you've ever written,' I told Pavel. 'I love it.'

He smiled. 'It's for you. It's what you wanted.' He quoted the last line of my *Stalin 2* article: *If Lupus ever makes a film set in a madhouse, I can guess who they'll call.*

He and Thomas explained that this one had been tailored specifically to my darkest fantasies. The most bizarre and unexpected gift.

'Thanks,' I said. 'I think.'

After dinner Cameron and I walked back to our apartment. It was a chilly night but I was warm in my blue velvet dress. Going to Prague always feels like coming home and I carried my *pomlázky* with pride as we navigated the winding cobblestone streets. Cameron couldn't resist positioning me over a railing and giving me a few flicks with one of the braided whips. A group of boys nearby saw and cheered him on in Czech, making me blush.

He ran his hand up the inside of my thigh, making me shiver.

'When we get back to the apartment,' he said, 'we can rehearse the rape scene.'

'Mmmm . . . I'd hate that very much.'

28. STALIN 3: THE MADHOUSE

I didn't have to be at the studio until late afternoon the next day, to shoot the hostage exchange. So we stayed up late. Cameron tied me to the bed and did terrible things to me, threatening to send me to the punishment room if I struggled. Actually, he didn't hurt me at all. But he's so very good at threatening.

Afterwards we went through the script, drinking *slivovice* and talking about the story. Cameron helped me run my lines and I studied the notes I had made to go with the out-of-sequence shooting schedule. Shooting the final scene first was going to be disorienting.

When we arrived at the studio the next day, they set about transforming me into a madhouse inmate. Irena dressed me in an old brown 1950s dress with a threadbare cardigan and clumpy boots. Magda smeared gunk in my hair and smudged grey under my eyes to give me a hollow, haunted expression. I looked like a refugee who'd been through hell. As Nikolaja had.

The hostage exchange takes place on an abandoned railway bridge. A near-deserted cycle track runs alongside the line. Decades of soot and oil have stained the gravel between the tracks. It's a desolate location and Zbyšek was hoping for rain. He got his wish. The atmosphere couldn't have been better. It was a cold, bleak evening with a leaden sky and a fine, misty rain.

Zbyšek told me to get into character, to remember everything that had gone before that led up to this moment. Nikolaja has no idea she is being released; she thinks they are taking her out to shoot her. But by this time she no longer cares.

The shot looks like archive footage until the grainy black and white turns to colour and the camera zooms in to show Nikolaja and her captors waiting to make the exchange.

We must have been a strange sight to passing motorists: two men in leather Gestapo-style trench coats, another in a West German military uniform and a miserable-looking refugee girl. Together with a film crew. And as our little party walked to the bridge Cameron did his hardest job yet. He played the voice of my conscience, telling me all the terrible things Nikolaja would be saying to herself. Everyone else was laughing and joking, and that only made me feel more isolated.

'You betrayed Libuše,' Cameron hissed in my ear, making me flinch. 'Your only friend. She'll never forgive you.'

My eyes filled with tears as I embraced the guilt, letting myself believe I really had betrayed her. It was bitterly cold in the drizzle and I shivered, clutching the dirty sweater around me and refusing the offer of a coat. It could only help my headspace to be miserable.

'Laudon's daughter,' Cameron said with disgust. 'Your father would be ashamed to see you now.'

I thought of my own father to make it real. Cameron's words bored into me like a corkscrew and I called myself the one word he didn't: coward.

My eyes were like stones as the Czech agents shoved me forward and I began to stumble along the bridge. I stared into the distance and beyond it. Racked with guilt, I was both apathetic and afraid. I didn't even look at Pavel as I passed him on the bridge. Two men were waiting for me on the other side – one in a military uniform and the other in a raincoat.

As I got closer the man in the raincoat spoke to me: 'It's over now, *Fräulein*,' he said in German with a fatherly smile. 'You're safe.'

He motioned to his companion, who removed his jacket and put it around my shoulders. The simple kindness was too much for me. I broke down, sobbing convulsively, startled by the intensity of my reaction.

And that was just the first scene.

The next day we shot the corridor and shower scenes at the madhouse. Lupus had rented an old gymnasium with wire mesh changing rooms and a frightening communal shower with broken taps and chipped tiles. It was straight out of a horror movie.

Alexandra Wolf played the corpse. Not a demanding role unless you consider that she spent two hours in makeup while Magda applied the gunshot wound to her back and the rest of the day lying uncomfortably on her stomach on a stretcher so as not to disturb it. There's no Academy Awards ceremony for CP films, but if there were, Magda would definitely win the Oscar for Best Makeup Effects.

I had met one of my fellow inmates the night before, in the studio. Her name was Sara Vojtisková. She was cast as Eliška, who freaks out in the day room and has to be put in a straitjacket after a cold shower. This was her first film for Lupus. I shook my head in bewilderment. There had been some consolation in *Stalin 2* knowing that all the victims were actual Scene players, so I didn't worry that anything would be too much for them. But this one had two newcomers.

As it turned out, the girl who was to play Libuše was ill and had to cancel. So they gave the role to Sara. And some of it *was* too much for her.

Throughout the shoot I kept asking myself who on earth would find the story arousing. Would anyone? *Should* anyone? If this was an outsider's glimpse into my fantasies, what did that say about me? The madhouse was an ideal setting for the abusive power dynamic and the anti-Communist theme gave the story a dramatic edge. It was undeniably powerful, but it seemed almost a shame to waste such a story on a CP film.

It wasn't difficult to get back into Nikolaja's headspace. Only this time I had to go deeper; I had to be broken. I had no idea how it would feel and I was surprised at how comfortable it was. It was a very childlike state. All my stubbornness and indignation from *Stalin 2* were gone and in their place were total resignation and surrender.

I thought of the Stanford Prison Experiment, where the 'guards' and 'prisoners' so internalised their roles that the experiment took on a life of its own. It got out of hand in only six days, leaving 'prisoners' emotionally scarred and 'guards' shaken by their sadistic behaviour.

The power of roleplay lies in its ability to blur the lines between reality and fantasy. It allows you to get inside someone else's skin and live their life for a short while. It's not acting; it's *experiencing*. I've always felt compelled to explore and experience the darker side of life. I want to feel the emotional pain as I do the physical, to absorb it and understand it. Most of all I want to return from the experience, alive, enriched and empowered. A survivor.

Libuše's suicide was the hardest scene. The girls filed into the shower, still bedraggled from earlier shower scenes. The guards turned the hose on us and we shrieked at the blast of cold water, trying to avoid the spray. It was my third dose of cold water that day. Libuše slipped behind the rest of us and when she was out of sight of the camera, they cut the shot and it was time to make her up.

Again, Magda did an amazing job and the result was startlingly realistic. Libuše lay on the wet floor of the shower with her arm out to the side. Magda poured fake blood on the wound and it ran down onto the tiles, staining the water and swirling down the drain.

Once the cameras were rolling, the line of girls parted and we screamed as we saw what had happened. I ran to Libuše, crying and begging her to wake up. She was dead because of me, because she couldn't live with the shame of what I had done. I turned on the guards, screaming, 'Murderers! Murderers!'

After the suicide scene, the rest of the cast was free to leave. I had to go back to the studio to shoot the narration. I noticed Sara by herself in the shower, tearfully scrubbing at the glue and fake blood on her wrist. Startled and concerned, I stayed behind. She offered me a brave smile, but it was clear that it had disturbed her. It suddenly occurred to me how bizarre all this must seem to an outsider. I could imagine the same thing happening on the set of a horror film. The cast and crew joking and horsing around – 'Right, that's one murder done! Next victim!' – and a newbie actress haunted by the blood and gore.

Critics argue that realistic drama has no place in an erotic film. But they're missing the point. The dramatic scenes are elements of plot and character, not erotica. Libuše's suicide is not meant to turn you on; it's meant to make you empathise with the girls. Just as some comedies make you cry and some dramas have elements of comic relief, erotic films can have important things to say.

The scene was painful for Sara, which made it painful for me. Her horror at the blood added to Nikolaja's sense of guilt. It made Libuše seem even more fragile. I heard my old drama teacher, Mr Wynn, saying, 'Use it!' And I did.

I had to go forward in time now, to record Nikolaja's 'statement'. Back at the studio they effected another transformation – from dishevelled inmate to forlorn young woman. It was ten years later, so Magda gave me a 1960s bouffant hairdo. I was struck by how much I looked like old photographs of my mother.

Recounting everything in a flat beaten voice, Nikolaja gazes into the distance with haunted eyes, remembering, reliving.

I was dreading the narration about Libuše. One line was so poignant it had made me cry when I first read the script. Now I had to try and say it with the weight of Nikolaja's memories behind it.

I saw Sara abandoned in the shower, scrubbing away her death. My throat clenched. 'You know, Libuše was the only person who had smiled at me in all those years . . .'

I kept expecting to run out of tears, but it just didn't happen.

29. BE CAREFUL WHAT YOU WISH FOR

Rape. The most dangerous fantasy of all and yet the most common.

In the original version of the script, only Libuše was raped (and off-screen at that). I jokingly said I was disappointed that it wasn't Nikolaja. Two days later, Pavel had written a new scene just for me. And this one was to be on camera. I think my rapist (Lukaš Wolf) was more disturbed by it than I was.

After the guards abuse Libuše and toss her back into the top bunk they untie Nikolaja and drag her out of the lower bunk. One of the guards shoves his hand down her pants. 'She's wet!' he exclaims.

Cut to Nikolaja in the studio, reliving the moment as she records her statement: 'I didn't want it. I swear I didn't want it.'

The guards stand over their friend as he pins Nikolaja down on the floor and fucks her. Nikolaja is overwhelmed with shame, hating herself for the way her body responds. But she's learned not to fight, so she surrenders to it. What Libuše sees is a little whore enjoying it.

Zbyšek said the scene would only be a close-up of my face, shot from over Lukaš's shoulder. The script says that Nikolaja doesn't resist, but I didn't know what to do. When you're playing with emotions like that, you have to *feel* them to portray them convincingly. Blur the lines. I'd learned in drama school that, if you were 'honest', the emotions would come naturally. Let go, lose control and let it happen.

There was no rehearsal; we just started. Lukaš pinned my wrists down and I was instantly there. I imagined all the abuse Nikolaja had experienced and witnessed. And even though Libuše was watching, I didn't have the courage to resist. I would do anything to avoid the torment she had endured. If that meant being their whore, so be it.

The carpet was rough beneath me, like sandpaper. Lukaš had no idea how much it was hurting me and I wasn't about to tell him. It helped me. I winced every time the abrasive threads ground into me and I looked at Lukaš's face, willing Nikolaja to see a lover instead of a rapist. When she began to feel pleasure, Nikolaja pushed aside the shame and embraced the fantasy. It wasn't brave, but it protected her.

At last it was time for the scene I was really dreading. The guards left me on the floor, my pyjama bottoms down and my shirt torn open. Crying and ashamed, I got shakily to my feet. Libuše was lying on her side, gazing at me, and I put my face close to hers.

Sara has extraordinarily expressive eyes and she stared at me while I reached for her hand.

'I'm sorry,' I whispered. 'I'm so sorry.'

Her beautiful eyes turned cold and dead, like the eyes a doll. She pulled her hand from mine and turned away.

This time I *did* need comforting.

The shoot was over, but I couldn't get out of Nikolaja's head. And the strange thing was that I didn't want to. Painful as that place was, I was comfortable there. There was an eerie serenity in such total helplessness. It was an extreme I'd longed to experience. I lived it for days. I even dreamed about it.

Adele told me, 'Lupus have gone beyond the spanking genre into the mindfuck genre.' Yes, the mindfuck is definitely at the core of my kink. I'm not a physical masochist, but I think I've learnt that I'm a psychological one. I was more deeply in the headspace than I ever expected to be on camera.

I missed the madhouse desperately. There's always a feeling of melancholy at the end of a shoot, but this was more like Stockholm Syndrome. I felt threatened by the thought of leaving my dark little shell. Returning to reality would mean taking control again and that was frightening after being so completely dependent.

The day after the shooting wrapped, I spotted two policemen in the Prague Metro and I instantly felt a rush of fear at the sight of the uniforms. The feeling was unsettling, but I was thrilled that I had internalised Nikolaja's experience to such a degree. Not all emotional scars are bad.

I kept the pyjamas. Sometimes I still wear them.

Yahoo! groups: nikiflynn

The spanker in the new homepage pic looks like he'd rather be doing something else, Niki. I've never seen such a lacklustre pose. Is he examining his nails or suffering hypoxia?

Father Jon, Canberra

Aw, come on – we all take pictures that aren't brilliant. You should see the ones of me I *don't* post!

Love,
Niki

E X A C T L Y!!!!!

Finally, the *real* Niki! We've all obviously obsessed over the superior quality material – what must we do to get a glimpse into the honest-to-goodness/behind-the-scenes reality?

Sidney, Los Angeles

30. A SLAP IN THE FACE

'Woodley!' I bark, charging into Samantha's room. 'You said you'd do that essay.'

'Well, maybe you should be doing your *own* homework.'

'You said you'd do it,' I growl, giving her a vicious shove.

'Don't push me!' Samantha pushes me back and we wrestle on the bed, our red tartan skirts flipping up to flash our white school knickers. Samantha winds up on the floor and I stand over her threateningly.

'Get up.'

She scrambles to her feet, glaring at me.

'Let's take it outside,' I say.

'No, let's do it right here.'

'Fine, let's—'

SLAP!

The blow spins me around and I fall back on the bed, stunned, my face stinging. I leap at her and we tussle until Gillian Lancer arrives.

'What's going on here?' she demands.

'She started it!'

'No, *she* started it!'

Our housemistress is scandalised. 'Young ladies don't conduct themselves in that manner in my school! Goodness gracious! Rolling around, showing your knickers . . . You're like a couple of hoodlums.'

'I had to defend myself,' Samantha blurts out. 'She came barging into my room—'

'Well, she was supposed to do something and she didn't and she doesn't keep her word—'

'Oh yeah, I was supposed to do *her homework* for her—'

'Liar! You were *not*!'

We stop squabbling when we notice the chilly silence.

'Sorry?' Gillian asks sweetly, waiting to hear the rest of the story.

I met Samantha Woodley when David Pierson wrote to tell me there was an American spanking model languishing in England with no kinky friends to hang out with. The doe-eyed California girl had starred in several Shadow Lane films and was a regular on the Firm Hand Spanking website. Cameron and I got together with her and her boyfriend for a weekend of roleplay that left us hungry for more. 'More' became a 24-part series called 'English School'.

I'd done two more shoots with SOL after the Great American Girl Project, working with veteran top Gillian Lancer. These were purely school-themed scenarios with none of the squicky stuff I'd disliked on their first shoot. Gillian runs a school in West Yorkshire for adults who want a taste of real English discipline. In her role as Miss Hastings-Gore, she's the perfect no-nonsense schoolmistress. She instantly became one of my favourite tops.

One of those SOL scenes had been particularly difficult for both of us – not because of the severity, but rather the lack thereof. The director wanted a very mild scene. Gillian's used to dealing with men, so she's not accustomed to holding back. And I'm no good at faking that it hurts when it doesn't. I felt ridiculous yelping and kicking over her lap while she barely turned my cheeks pink. When it was over we both sighed with relief.

'Thank God that's over,' I said. 'That was *hard*!' Gillian echoed the sentiment.

The director was baffled. 'What do you mean? She was barely even touching you.'

Moral: You can go easy on the vanilla girls, but don't cheat the real enthusiasts.

Firm Hand promises 'Beautiful girls, painful punishments', so, when they asked me if I knew anyone who could handle the two of us, I suggested Gillian.

The American brats arrived at their English boarding school in tight jeans and skimpy tops. Full of attitude and bravado, we sneered at the rules and the uniforms. We complained that the shirt collars were too tight and that the skirts made us look fat. Gillian took us in hand immediately, giving us each a hard over-the-knee spanking.

Samantha and I had an easy chemistry and the three of us played off each other well. We all had fun as the series progressed. Shooting sequences like this is an exhausting process – far more demanding than a movie. A Lupus caning may be severe, but it's over in a couple of minutes. A website shoot requires several separate punishment scenes with a variety of implements.

In the next scene Samantha and I found a small wooden paddle in the classroom, which we broke in an act of defiance. Actually, Cameron had discovered it in the bin while the director was setting up for the shoot. Gillian had broken it on a 'schoolboy' the day before and thrown it away. But we thought it would make a great prop and a perfect excuse for punishment, so Cameron fished it out of the bin and stuck it back together with Blu-Tack.

Alone in the room, with Miss Hastings-Gore nowhere in sight, Samantha and I investigated the implements on display. I picked up a leather tawse and slapped it against my hand, wincing at the sting.

'She is *not* hitting me with that,' I declared.

Samantha grabbed the paddle. 'Look at this one – it's like a 2×4!' She slammed it down on the desk. But, instead of breaking in half like it was supposed to, it slowly peeled apart along the Blu-Tack seam, one half hanging by the putty strips as though attached with chewing gum. We burst out laughing.

Cameron stuck it back together for another take. This time Samantha landed the blow on the edge of the desk, parallel with the break. The thing split in two lengthwise and the smaller piece flew up, twirling in the air in front of us. Brilliant! Gillian came running to see what we'd done. And since our hands had committed the crime, our hands paid the price. Two strokes of the tawse on each palm.

I hate hand punishments, but it had never been done before on Firm Hand, so I was game. It hurt terribly, but the noise wasn't that loud. Cameron graciously offered his own palms to Gillian for sound dubbing.

Next came the ruler for passing notes in class. Then the cane for trying to escape. That scene's got a great exterior shot – two schoolgirls lowering a rope down to the street twenty feet below.

Gym class – the paddle. Improper uniform – the slipper. Smuggling alcohol into our room – the hairbrush. By the end of the first day we were very tender. We'd written all the scenarios in advance, pacing ourselves by building up to the worst implements after warming up with the lighter ones.

The second day started with my favourite scene of all: the catfight. I wanted it to be more than just half-hearted scuffling, so I told Samantha to slap me.

'I can't do that!'

'Yes, you can. Trust me, the guys will love it.'

We choreographed our little dance. I'd push her, she'd push me back and when I retaliated, she'd slap me. Then the fight would begin in earnest and Gillian would break it up. We did the opening argument, which led to some shoving. But she forgot to slap me. So we cut and picked up where we'd left off.

'Let's take it outside,' I said, trying to provoke her.

'No, I want to do it right here.' Samantha grabbed my arms and spun me around. I stumbled and fell to the floor and we cracked up. Lame.

We tried again and this time she remembered. By then I'd completely forgotten about the slap and it caught me off guard. It took me a moment to realise what had happened and Samantha looked worried that she'd hurt me. But I snapped out of it and lunged for her, pulling her hair and making her cry out. She pushed me down over the bed and we scuffled until Gillian arrived and got the truth out of Samantha.

'Niki's been bullying me into doing her homework and she was really pissed off that I—'

Gillian's eyes widened. '*Pardon?*'

'Sorry. I mean she was really . . . upset.'

'I see. So we have one girl who's a bully and another who swears like a navvy.'

'She hit me,' I said, pointing to my cheek. 'See?'

'Dear me, that does look red and sore,' she agreed and turned to Samantha. 'You did that?'

'Yes, but she came in first and I had to defend myself!'

'You invited me in,' I said with a wounded look.

'I wouldn't invite you anywhere.'

Gillian gave us an icy smile. 'Oh, well, I'll invite you some-where, girls. I'll invite you to raise your skirts and drop your knickers.'

Touché.

Samantha went first, touching her toes for twelve strokes of the cane. She hates the cane, so we'd agreed beforehand that I'd get it worse. I was to get eighteen. In exchange, she said she'd take it harder with an implement *I* hated.

Afterwards, she stood in front of the door with me. This was where the director wanted to cut the scene. Part two would be my caning. He asked for some kind of parting shot from us to round off the sequence.

Forgetting which of us had just been caned, Samantha said, 'You got exactly what you deserved,' and crossed her arms in smug satisfaction. She leaned back against the door, which promptly fell open, spilling her into Gillian's office.

I never imagined that viewers would be interested in the outtakes, but they're immensely popular. Some of my fans enjoy them more than the actual scenes. They say it's nice to be reassured that there's fun and games behind the drama.

I just happened to be browsing the web . . . and waxing nostalgic . . . when it suddenly occurred to me . . . I have not seen my favorite spanking model in a while!! She's not only missing from the SOL website, but she's nowhere to be found on the other six UK spanking websites I regularly subscribe to.

So, what better way to get 'to the bottom' of the issue (pun intended) than to go to the source.

Niki Flynn . . . where are you? And why are we not seeing MORE of you? Please don't break my heart and tell me you have 'retired' from the scene! Perish the thought!

An avid fan who loves his Niki

31. THE CAGE

I had shot two movies for Strictly English, one of the oldest CP film companies in the UK. My third shoot fell through. It was an elaborate story about a girl and her unscrupulous therapist. He plants the hypnotic suggestion that she behave like a petulant child and throw a tantrum whenever she doesn't get her way. Her uncle then has carte blanche to *treat* her like a child. I was looking forward to it, but the director had to cancel because of illness.

Cameron and I had set the whole weekend aside to go down south for it. Shoots also offered an excuse for a road trip, a chance to explore castles and stately homes. We felt cheated of both kink and culture. So I dug around on the net in search of action. Sure enough, there was a dungeon in Manchester hosting a Back to School party that Saturday. There were pictures of the playspace on the website. It was a proper dungeon, kitted out with lots of devices we never got to play with, including a pillory and a Catherine wheel. I wrote to request an invitation and we had our weekend set. We were off to Manchester a few days later.

We followed the directions to a railway arch in a run-down part of town. There was no car park, so we left the car on the street and just had to hope it would still be there when we returned. It reminded me of some of the clubs I'd gone to when I lived in New York.

We were dressed for a CP party, me in my Japanese school uniform and Cameron in his headmaster's gown. But despite the school theme, most people were in leather, latex and PVC. While BDSM and CP do overlap, the two scenes differ enormously. BDSM tends to be more overtly sexual, for a start. We didn't have much experience in the BDSM scene, and I was genuinely surprised to see people having sex on some of the equipment. You'd be thrown out of most spanking parties for that.

Cameron directed me to the leather whipping bench in the middle of the room. Built specially for kneeling on and bending right over, it had leather straps to hold every part of me in place: wrists, ankles, elbows, knees, back. I couldn't move at all and I felt my body responding. He gave me a light spanking and caning, but I knew it was just a warm-up. We had the whole night.

Cameron struck up a conversation with Lisa, a curvy redhead in an elegant tight-laced corset. Her Scottish boyfriend Ewan was wearing a latex kilt with all the accoutrements – also latex. Nothing underneath. They were hardcore exhibitionists and after making noisy use of the sex sling in the far corner, they moved on to the Catherine Wheel. Ewan strapped Lisa in and spun her around, fingering and licking her while she was upside-down and inviting others to assist him. I'd tried the wheel earlier, amazed at the number of straps and buckles and harnesses. It was like a fairground ride, but the security was necessary if you wanted it to hold someone upside-down. Cameron had molested me a bit, but nothing like what Ewan was doing to Lisa. I felt a little out of my depth in my school uniform and schoolgirl panties.

They joined us again afterwards. Lisa was buzzing from the experience. There was a whispered exchange between Cameron and Ewan and then Cameron said, 'It's time.'

I blushed and looked at the floor. I knew what he meant. For days he'd been telling me about the 'grope cage' pictured on the website. It didn't look like much in the photo – just a tall black box like a coffin standing on end. In reality it was a cage covered with black cloth. The cloth had holes in various places, just big enough for arms to reach through.

Cameron asked Ewan for his help and the two of them led me into the back room. I'd been fantasising about it too, but now that it was about to happen I felt like backing out. Especially when Cameron took a length of rope out of his pocket.

'Take off your bra and panties,' he said.

I hesitated.

'If you'd rather be whipped first, that can be arranged.'

Several people were watching with interest. I felt like a diver entering a shark cage while dorsal fins scythed through the water all around me.

I obeyed and Cameron tied my wrists together, securing them over my head inside the cage. My heart began to pound. The door swung shut with a metal clang and I panted in the dark, waiting.

A pair of hands emerged from the cloth in front of me. I closed my eyes as they found my shirt and reached up under it, squeezing my breasts. I had no idea who it was. Another pair of hands groped behind me, fondling my bottom through my skirt before flipping it up to pinch my cheeks. I twisted and squirmed, but I only had about a foot to spare around me. There was no way to escape the molestation. If I pressed myself against the bars, I would only make myself more accessible to the people on the other side.

I was sure one pair of hands must be Cameron's and the other Ewan's, though I couldn't guess which was which. Neither touch seemed familiar. Before long there was a fifth hand somewhere to my left, stroking my thigh. I shivered as the fingers crept up underneath the front of my skirt. Soft feminine fingers stroked my face from the right and I sighed as she ran her nails up and down the back of my neck, giving me gooseflesh. Lisa? Someone else? I didn't know who any of my tormentors were and I kept my eyes closed to keep it that way.

The male hand under my skirt was getting very intimate and I jumped as the palm pressed up against me, cupping me firmly and forcing me up on tiptoe. I arched into his touch, my sex throbbing. Then he released me and his fingers stroked my labia. Other hands whispered through the slits in the fabric and held me firmly in place whenever I struggled. I was overwhelmed with sensations as strangers played with me – tickling, teasing, tormenting.

The first pair of hands began to pinch my nipples, rolling them between fingers and thumbs. I gasped and whimpered, nearing overload as the fingers between my legs demanded entrance. I agonised for a moment whether or not to allow it, but then my resolve melted and I surrendered.

I was at the mercy of a dozen hands and once I was freed from the cage I would have no idea who had done what. For all I knew it was Cameron who was stroking my wetness with such insistence. But I suspected it wasn't. I gave a little cry as the invading finger pushed between my lips. I clamped my legs tightly around the hand, feeling violated and debauched, loving it.

Whoever was fondling my bottom began to smack me softly and the man on my left withdrew his finger and then plunged it into me again, rougher this time. I cried out and pulled at the ropes. The girl was stroking my hair, drawing her nails across my scalp and making me tingle. My whole body was vibrating. Greedily, I regretted that no one could get to my feet, as that probably would have sent me over the edge.

Finally, Cameron's voice cut through the confusion of hands molesting me. 'I think that's enough for now.' His voice held the promise of more later.

There was some soft male laughter and the hands slowly withdrew. Their reluctance was palpable. I heard the cage door rattle and suddenly I was more embarrassed by the prospect of being let out than of staying in and submitting to more groping. I kept my eyes shut tightly as Cameron untied me and led me out. I smoothed my skirt down, a feeble attempt to regain my modesty. My legs were trembling. I couldn't look at anyone. I covered my face and pressed myself close to Cameron, blushing to my toes.

He peeled my hands away from my face, grinning as he told me to look around the room and try and guess who had been doing what to me. Mortified, I buried my face again. People chuckled.

I suddenly thought of Victorian ladies who used to say they thought they would die of shame. I know exactly what they were talking about, even if they probably hadn't got as much pleasure out of that shame as I had.

Are you the actress who has her hair cut short in the movie Crime and Punishment?

I noticed in your website gallery that you have many different hairstyles – have you done any other haircutting videos I might be able to find? And what in the world inspired you to cut your hair for the video in the first place? May I ask what it was like?

Do you do custom videos for a proper fee?

Curious in America

32. IN GERMANY NO ONE CAN HEAR YOU SCREAM

Did I mention I have a thing for uniforms?

When German fetish photographer Ben Marcato asked me about my fantasies, I didn't hold back. I told him my darkest ones. Bondage. Interrogation. Uniforms. Boots. He loved it. He said he didn't often find girls willing to play so rough. Or rather – girls willing to be so roughly *played with*.

Ben proposed a shoot that sounded too good to be true. Three men in military uniforms would tie me up and manhandle me in gritty black and white photos. In Germany. How could I say no?

I had never done a straight photo shoot before; I'd only done stills to accompany spanking videos. They were fun, but never as exciting as roleplay. Posing for stills is a static process, with no psychological edge. But Ben was a genuine BDSM enthusiast and his emails led me to believe the shoot might be more than just the familiar pose-click-pose-click routine.

Cameron had a business trip in Germany, so we went over together by ferry and I peeled off to stay in Cologne while he attended to business. Ben's studio was on the outskirts of Dortmund, a short train ride away.

I had a lot of German correspondents on the spanking forums, so I had arranged to meet three of them there while I was in their country. Jack was the first. I met him the night before the shoot.

He came to my hotel room to fetch me and we went out for dinner. Afterwards we smuggled some beer up to the room. We talked long into the night, but we were both too shy to initiate play. (Damn!)

I met Tom the next day. He's a photojournalist and he wanted to interview me for a German BDSM magazine. He was the one who had put me in touch with Ben and he agreed to go to the shoot with me. He also met me in my room and we left together for the train station and got to know each other on the way to the studio.

The day after the shoot, Tom returned to do the interview in my hotel room, which lasted about an hour. I'm sure you can see where this is going.

Soon after he left, my third German friend, Ludwig, arrived and came straight up to my room. We hung out for a couple of hours and then went out for dinner. The whispered exchange between the guys at reception didn't need translating. Three different guys in as many nights. Ludwig suggested that he storm into the lobby shouting that the American whore in room 310 had stolen his wallet. I was all for it. I was still high from the shoot the day before and the public drama would have rounded off my Germany adventure perfectly. In the end, wiser judgment prevailed. Instead, we had a German lesson in my room that involved a cane and me counting to thirty. I imagined the desk clerks eavesdropping outside, exchanging startled expressions.

But back to the uniforms.

Ben took Tom and me to his office, a cramped space littered with photographic and lighting equipment. It betrayed no hint of what he was planning. I'd brought along a couple of outfits they could destroy: a gauzy white bridal negligee I used to dance in and a posh red dress I'd bought on eBay for the purpose.

'Are we shooting in here?' I asked doubtfully.

'No,' Ben said. 'The shoot will be . . . somewhere else.'

'Where?'

'Oh, you'll see.'

My stomach began to flutter.

Then two of my tormentors arrived. Ralf was a big muscular guy covered in tattoos, a local BDSM player. He was also a professional combat trainer and weapons expert. He brandished a fearsome military hunting knife and I trembled. Knives are a huge turn-on. The idea of being held at knifepoint by someone who knows how to use one properly is thrilling.

The second guy was Wolfgang. He was tall, lean and angular, and also a player. I was relieved they weren't just vanilla models with no clue about fetish stuff. That would have been awkward, but you don't feel like a freak among your own kind. With matching sadistic smiles they told me they were looking forward to playing with me.

'We have some surprises in store for you,' Wolfgang said.

I chewed my lip nervously and moved closer to Tom. He'd translated the model release for me earlier, joking that he was now my agent, so I'd come to think of him as my protector. 'Don't let them kill me,' I whispered.

'I won't,' he said. 'Not before I get my interview anyway.'

Ralf and Wolfgang started to get dressed and my pulse quickened as I saw what they were going to wear. Stasi uniforms. My face felt hot and I pressed my thighs together, squirming at the sight of the intimidating insignia. There's just something about a military uniform that commands immediate respect.

Ralf saw me watching and gave me a wicked grin, striking a pose in his flared army breeches and immaculately polished boots. 'It's very German, yes?'

Oh, yes. Very German indeed.

Once Ralf and Wolfgang were dressed, the four men gathered the equipment and abandoned me while they went to set up. I paced the room, mentally preparing myself. Ben had told me to choose some music and I was pleased to discover two Rammstein CDs on the shelf. I couldn't imagine a better soundtrack for a Stasi interrogation than Till Lindemann's deep guttural voice and rolled Rs.

I dug through my suitcase. I'd brought a ton of clothes and I finally settled on a short black dress with high heels. I wasn't sure how to do my makeup for black and white photos, so I stuck with what I usually used for colour shoots. I took my time getting ready, but there was still no sight of the men. By the time they came to get me, nearly an hour later, I had worked myself into a nervous frenzy.

'Are you ready?' Ben asked, grinning.

'I hope so.'

We crossed the street and entered an old warehouse. Ben took me by the hand and led me down two flights of cold concrete steps into a shadowy vestibule. I had no idea what to expect. A bunker? A slaughterhouse? He unlocked the door and I stepped inside. The empty space was cavernous. It looked like an abandoned factory. About 150 yards long, 15 yards wide and 20 feet high. Iron girders branched from the walls and ceiling, covered with twenty years' worth of dust.

On a raised platform at one end of the hall was a battered desk with an old-fashioned gooseneck lamp on one corner and straight-backed chairs on either side. Lights and reflectors lined the periphery, spotlighting the area. Ralf appeared beside me and I jumped. With an amused chuckle he displayed a pair of handcuffs, then grabbed my wrists and locked them together behind my back. The opening bars of '*Reise, Reise*' begin to pound from the CD player and Ralf dragged me into the light.

Wolfgang sat behind the desk, watching me from under the rim of his peaked cap. With a snarl, Ralf shoved me down in the chair across from his companion.

'*Wirst du uns sagen, was wir wissen möchten?*' Wolfgang asked pleasantly.

I melted at his crisp pronunciation. Was I going to tell them what they wanted to know? This was an unexpected treat; I hadn't anticipated an actual roleplay! I shook my head helplessly. 'I don't understand,' I pleaded, instantly disengaging from the real world and losing myself in the fantasy. '*Ich verstehe Sie nicht!*'

My interrogators laughed coldly and Wolfgang tilted the lamp to shine it in my face. I squinted in the harsh light and turned away, but Ralf fisted a hand in my hair and yanked my head back up. With slow deliberation, Wolfgang got up, standing over me threateningly. He lifted my chin and peered into my face.

'*Ja, auch dich werden wir zum Reden bringen.*'

I glared at him in defiance, my heart pounding. 'I won't tell you a thing!'

English has no familiar form of 'you' and it's a subtle but significant void. The forced intimacy of an abusive official assuming the familiar *du* is a vulgar affront. It's belittling. Especially when you know *you're* expected to use the formal *Sie*. You can imagine what it does to me.

Wolfgang's eyes narrowed and he struck the desk with his fist. '*Reden!*'

I flinched and Ralf shoved me forward, pushing me down over the desk. A hand connected sharply with my thigh and I yelped in surprise. We hadn't negotiated any limits and I found the presumption exhilarating.

I struggled, bruising my wrists. It was only then that I noticed Ben taking pictures. I'd forgotten him completely!

Wolfgang bent me forward over the desk on my stomach with my head turned to the side. He held me down with my cheek pressing into the scarred wood. Ralf grabbed one of my shoes and raised it above my head, as though about to stab me with the stiletto heel. I played along, pretending terror. Wolfgang shouted at me again and again to talk, startling me when I wasn't expecting it. Through it all Rammstein echoed off the walls, cocooning me in a pocket of primal energy that was like a psychic vibrator, bombarding me with stimuli in all the right ways.

I found some pluck when they pinned me down on my back. I braced my bare feet against Ralf's chest, pushing hard against him and making him work to keep me in position. Then I put my heel against his jaw and he mimed the pain of having been kicked. Then anger and retaliation. It was brilliant.

They continued to mistreat me, slapping my bottom and pulling my hair while I resisted and tried to get away. Then they blindfolded me and one held me down while the other planted his boot on the back of my neck. When they hauled me up again it was to tear open my dress and maul my breasts. I wasn't wearing one of the disposable dresses, but at that point I didn't care. I fought back, losing every time and adoring being overpowered.

After what felt like an hour, a distant voice said something in German and the music stopped. The hands around my arms and throat relaxed. A break. I drifted back to reality. There was a friendly squeeze and someone asked if I was OK.

I nodded drunkenly. 'Uh-huh.'

'Is it too much?'

'Uh-uh.'

Ralf unlocked me and I rubbed my wrists. They were red and chafed and I knew I'd have some dramatic bruises to show for it. Lucky for me it was autumn; long sleeves would hide the marks from vanilla eyes.

'Great stuff, Niki!' Ben enthused, offering me a bottle of champagne. There were no glasses, so we passed the bottle around, joking that we should include some of our photos in tourist brochures: 'Come visit friendly Deutschland!'

'How did it look?' I asked Tom.

'Intense,' he said, impressed. He'd had no idea what to expect either. He photographed us all goofing around and his behind-the-scenes images are great. Right after the scene, Wolfgang gave me a fierce hug and Tom caught it on film. It's one of my all-time favourite pictures; I don't think I've ever seen myself look happier.

It was time to go back to work. I changed into a different dress and prepared for more abuse. Ben rearranged the lights and reflectors while Wolfgang tied my wrists to an iron beam against the wall. His rough hands were all over me even before Ben had started photographing us. But I wasn't about to stop him. I was thoroughly enjoying myself. I twisted and struggled, relishing my helplessness and Wolfgang's aggressiveness. He lifted me from the hips like a dancer, forcing me to straddle him. It was like enacting a rape fantasy. He attacked me with gusto, thrusting against me with all the vigour of a conquering army, growling to me in English.

'*Sag es auf Deutsch*,' I whispered, blushing.

He was happy to accommodate me, switching to German and saying nasty things I didn't always understand. My knickers were soaked.

He shoved me back against the wall and tore my dress open at the front, exposing me. The iron girders and walls were filthy, covered with layers of dust and cobwebs. Every time he pressed me against the wall, dirt rubbed off on me. Wolfgang noticed and smiled. He ran his hand along the girder and then smeared it across my face and throat.

'*Schmutziges Mädchen*,' he said. Dirty girl.

The third villain arrived while we ate lunch. Dave was striking, with sharp vampiric cheekbones and piercing grey eyes. In his army fatigues and combat boots he was quite a contrast to my Stasi officers.

'Rammstein?' he exclaimed in dismay. 'Can't we listen to Johnny Cash instead?'

Fortunately, Ben said the model got to choose the music, so Till Lindemann growled '*Spiel Mit Mir*' while Wolfgang duct-taped my wrists together and looped them over the giant hook of an engine hoist. They raised the hook until I was standing on tiptoe. In my white Giselle gown and ballet slippers I was the picture of innocence waiting to be defiled. The men circled me like wolves and I squeezed my legs together in anticipation.

Ralf held the knife up in front of my face and I trembled, frightened and aroused. Then he slashed the flimsy dress to shreds, stuffing a handful of the material into my mouth to gag me. Dave lashed me with a small riding whip and I kicked and struggled to get free. But I was held fast.

I was lost in the moment and it was some time before I realised that I couldn't feel my hands any more. I spoke up and they instantly lowered the hook. The tape itself wasn't actually very tight, but the demi-pointe suspension had put a lot of pressure on my wrists. Once I was off the hook, the blood flow started returning and the pins and needles hurt more than the whipping had. Ben grabbed the EMT scissors they had on hand and started to cut through the tape. Unfortunately, it had been wrapped so many times around my wrists that the scissors couldn't get through it.

Ralf finally had to use his knife to get it off and the men took turns massaging my wrists back to life. Frustrated, I assured them that I just needed a little break, that they could put me back up there. But they weren't having it. It's something that happens when you're deep in a submissive headspace: your judgement becomes questionable and you're even more reliant on the dominant to take care of you. I was lucky to be in the hands of such responsible sadists.

Once my wrists returned to normal it was back to the interrogation desk for me. This time they blindfolded me, sat me down and taped my wrists to the sides of the chair. Then they set about scaring me. *Really* scaring me. They pounded on the desk, shouted at me and tilted the chair back as if they were going to let me fall.

Like pain, that kind of fear isn't erotic in the moment. But the adrenalin rush triggers a heightened state of both terror and elation. Every sensation feels like survival.

I was shaking and very near tears when a disturbing thought came to me. No one knew where I was. Not even Cameron. I was completely at the mercy of five self-proclaimed sadists I'd only met that morning. I was outnumbered, bound and blindfolded. The movie *Hostel* sprang to mind.

In the movie, unsuspecting tourists are lured to a hostel in Bratislava. It's a front for a human trafficking operation that provides victims for its elite members to torture and kill.

For a few moments I was truly terrified.

Then there was an ominous 'thump' as they set something on the desk in front of me. I was meant to hear it and I knew it was something awful. Someone got behind me and pushed me forwards, shoving my face close to the desk. I resisted, not knowing what was there. And when they pulled the blindfold off, my stomach twisted. Inches from my face was a plate seething with bloodworms.

They didn't stop there. Dave scooped up a handful of the tiny red squirming creatures, dropping several of them onto his tongue. Then he drew me close as if to kiss me and I clamped my mouth shut as tight as I could.

Behind me Ralf laughed, plucking a worm from the dish and holding it above my bare legs.

'*Nein! Nein!*' I screamed, panicking at the thought of it touching me.

Snakes, rats or spiders would have been no problem, but the nasty little writhing things filled me with horror. My heart was pounding so hard I thought it was going to explode. The few minutes they terrorised me seemed to last hours.

But my friendly abusers soon took pity on me. I sagged in my bonds with immense relief when they took the worms away and everyone was highly amused that I'd been so freaked out. I was surprised too; I never knew I had a worm phobia.

They blindfolded me again for the last session and I knew this was the one they'd been building up to. I told myself it couldn't possibly be worse than the worms.

I wore the disposable red dress and Ralf tied me to a pipe jutting from the wall. He menaced me with a straight razor, slicing the dress to ribbons and leaving me naked against the filthy wall.

There were footsteps all around me. Whispering. The sound of something heavy being dragged across the concrete floor. Something metal. I tensed in anticipation, having no idea what to expect. The dread was exhilarating.

All at once a loud WHOOSH! made me jump. There was the sensation of intense heat on my legs, as though I was standing next to a blast furnace. I pressed myself as close to the wall as I could, unable to stop thinking about *Hostel*. Had they paid someone for the privilege of burning me at the stake?

Another surge of heat flashed past my shoulder and I cried out, disoriented. I had no idea where the flames were or where I would feel their heat next.

Ralf laughed cruelly. 'Scream, girl. No one can hear you.'

The furnace roared again and all of a sudden there was a bright sharp burning sensation against my thigh and I yanked frantically at the ropes, crying.

'That's right,' Ralf growled. 'Smell the burning flesh.'

I sniffed and caught the smell of singed meat. Before I could process it there was another hot blast that made me yelp in terror.

This time the scorching sensation was on my lower back and again I smelled meat cooking as I jumped and twisted around, begging them not to hurt me. But I realised even as I was pleading that I wasn't burned at all.

A few seconds later someone pulled the blindfold off and I had to admire the mindfuck. Ralf had a propane torch in one hand and a chunk of meat on a hook in the other. And Dave was holding a Popsicle. Ralf grinned as he blasted the steak with the torch and Dave pressed the Popsicle against my ribs. It's one of the oldest tricks in the S&M book. If you're expecting fire, ice feels just like it.

In the end they didn't kill me. But they left me with the fondest memories I have of any shoot – film or photos. The intensity has never been matched.

The shoot had lasted seven hours and it was past midnight. Tom and I had missed the last train to Cologne, so Ben offered to drive us back to our separate hotels. I was shattered. Bruised and beaten, chafed and sore. But I was wide awake for the drive – hurtling at 140 miles an hour down the Autobahn in Ben's Mercedes. Ben was wide awake too. Excited about the shoot and very keen on the possibility of another one. Every time he turned to talk to me in the passenger seat I tensed up, clutching the armrest and willing him to keep his eyes front as we rocketed past everything else on the road.

Sometime around 2 a.m., the American whore staggered into the hotel, filthy and dishevelled, while the guy at reception tried hard not to stare.

Dear Niki,

After a lot of deliberation I have arranged a 121 with Miss Gillian Lancer at Westgate Old School. To widen my horizons, so to speak. I have been a bit like a parrot in the past (ie, just talked about it).

I have suggested a few strokes on the hands with the tawse and to round the session off a real 'six of the best' with the school cane. I know you have worked with her and hold her in high esteem. Any advice?

You're a brave girl. I am terrified!!!!

Thanks,

Nervous Schoolboy, London

33. MUCH OF MADNESS AND MORE OF SIN

The client is tied up and blindfolded when I arrive. Suspended by his wrists in leather cuffs, he's wearing an elaborate rope bondage harness. Charlotte tugs on the chain between the nipple clamps and he winces. She and Tia have been torturing him for an hour.

'Come join the fun,' Charlotte purrs. She's a wicked little fetish kitten in her red leather bodysuit, black thigh boots and policeman's hat. Tia's her apprentice, a Spanish vision in lacy Frederick's of Hollywood lingerie. Sexy, but no dominatrix; someone needs to take her shopping. Still, her exotic looks have potential.

Charlotte removes the blindfold and our victim takes in my black latex corset as I walk towards him. There's a cock ring maintaining his erection and Tia flicks him cruelly with a riding crop. His cock hardens even more as he responds. I circle him, tracing the lovely red stripes on his back with my fingers. He moans as I draw my nails down his tight, muscular body.

'He says he isn't a masochist,' Charlotte tells me. 'But we think he's fibbing.'

I smile as I take the black candle from the table and hold it up to his face. The flame dances with the movement. His eyes widen slightly, more with arousal than fear. I raise the candle and tilt it so that the wax droplets land on his chest, one by one, speckling him with cloudy black spots. He hisses through his teeth, throwing his head back. Tia brings the riding crop down on his ass and he writhes, groaning.

Some time later we release him and Charlotte instructs him to get himself off. He lies on his back on the floor. I kick off my shoes and stand on his chest, using the suspension rig for balance. I press my bare feet into his face, telling him to lick my feet and toes. He obeys with hungry enthusiasm. When he comes at last, he does it with my toes in his mouth.

Our victim's name was Kyle. He lived on an Indian reservation in South Dakota, where he participated in pain rituals and rites of passage. Shamans and mystics have used pain to achieve rapturous states for centuries. And whatever you call it – flying, bliss, ecstasy, transcendence – spanking and BDSM can take you to the same place. I've been there. On both sides.

I met Ava Taurel in New York City, long before I was a spanking model. I was interested in being a pro submissive in her dungeon. Ava was in her fifties but still sexy. Her patrician features gave her a regal appearance, though she was always a little offbeat. Flamboyant and eccentric the way only celebrities and drag queens are allowed to be.

She founded the Taurel Institute for Psychosexual Counselling, which was basically a dungeon tucked away inside a bland office building in midtown Manhattan. The daughter of a Russian prince and a Norwegian sculptress, Ava had led an extraordinary life. After winning a beauty contest at the Cannes Film Festival in 1960, she won a small part in a film and began a long career in the public eye. Over the years she'd been a dancer at the Folies Bergère in Paris, a film star in Mexico, a freelance photographer and documentary filmmaker, a sex counsellor and a dominatrix. Years later, in 2006, I was stunned and saddened to learn that she'd drowned while swimming in Mexico.

After dinner and a long discussion with Ava, I decided that being a pro sub wasn't for me. I'd have to do too many scenes I wasn't into and I'd feel silly calling someone 'Master'. D/s wasn't really my kink. I was a spanko, pure and simple. A bottom, but not a submissive. Definitely not a slave.

Ava smiled knowingly. 'Then you will be a domme,' she said.

I thought she was joking. But what Ava wanted, Ava got.

My stripper days had taught me that some men did see a domme in me. I hadn't been able to take advantage of it at the strip club, but I was intrigued by the challenge of doing it at the Taurel Institute. Turning to Edgar Allan Poe for inspiration, I called myself Lady Ligeia.

I arrived for my first gig in a slutty black leather dress and heels. It was all I had that looked remotely toppish.

'No, no, no,' said Ava, waving her hands as though dismissing servants. 'You're not going clubbing!' She dug through a wardrobe filled with fetish odds and ends, finally producing a blue PVC catsuit with a broken zip. Good enough.

'What does he want me to do?'

'Dominate him,' she said as though it were that simple. For her it probably was.

I looked at my new self in the mirror, paralysed with stage fright.

I'd been to private parties in New York. I'd played extensively with kinky friends. And occasionally I'd topped someone. But this was different. This man, my first customer, was *paying* me to make his fantasy a reality. (Quite a lot, too, though I'd only see half the fee.) What if I got it wrong? What if I did something he didn't like? What if he didn't like *me*?

Ava laughed. 'My dear, he's far more nervous than you are.'

I tried to imagine how he must be feeling. Left to wait in the dungeon with canes, crops and whips hanging on the walls around him. Knowing that any moment an unknown dominatrix would walk through the door and toy with him for the next hour. Yes, in his shoes I'd be terrified.

I took a deep breath, trying to conjure the 'thrilling and enthralling eloquence' of my namesake. I could do this. I feigned confidence and threw open the door to make a grand entrance. Startled, the client sprang to his feet.

'Hello,' I said, trying to sound authoritarian. What I came up with was simply an older version of my stripper coquette voice. 'I'm Lady Ligeia.' (I'd always heard it pronounced lye-JEE-ah, but I made it sound French: le-ZHAY-ah.)

'Hi,' he said meekly, lowering his eyes. He was about my height, but in my five-inch stilettos I towered over him.

'And what would you like to do?' I asked.

'Well, I want you to be my teacher.'

Ah. Teacher. I was a bit overdressed.

'OK,' I said, encouraging him.

'But what I like is a bit weird,' he mumbled.

'Weird is good.'

'I used to pick on the other boys at school and . . . well, one time in the changing room I grabbed this boy's underpants and yanked them up hard into his crack.'

I bit back a smile. 'You gave him a wedgie?'

'Yeah.'

'Just one time?'

He blushed. 'Well, no, I liked it so I did it a lot. To all the younger boys.'

'And now you think it's only fair that someone does it to you.'

'Well . . .'

'Well *what*, boy?' I snapped, jumping straight into the scene. 'Do you think it's funny?'

'No,' he mumbled.

'No what?'

He blushed and looked down.

'No, *miss*,' I supplied.

'No, miss,' he echoed.

'I don't think it's a bit funny. I think it's bullying. And you're going to be punished for it.'

I watched him physically shrink in size as he regressed in age. He let himself go, trusting me completely. Hunching his shoulders, he stared miserably at the floor as I scolded him, keeping my voice low and insinuating. It was surprisingly easy. I knew all the right things to say; I'd heard the same things said to *me*.

I made him strip down to his Calvin Klein underpants. They looked new and expensive and I suspected he'd bought them just for the occasion.

'Now you can stand in the corner, young man,' I said, barely recognising my voice, 'while you think about what you did.'

I took great delight in shaming him. Standing right behind him, I took hold of the waistband of his underpants. A shudder ran through his body and I could feel his anticipation like electricity.

'Did you think it was funny?' I asked, giving the Calvins a gentle tug.

He gasped, hesitating. 'No,' he moaned at last.

I gave a little jerk. 'No? You didn't enjoy it? You're lying!'

'No, miss! I mean, yes, I did think it was funny, but I don't now!'

His frantic babbling was charming. And while I didn't have a wedgie fetish myself, I found myself getting increasingly aroused.

He'd given me the key to his sexuality – the power to manipulate him completely. I loved it.

'You thought it was fun to humiliate the other boys,' I said softly. 'So it's only fair you know how it feels.' His erection tautened his underpants and I gave them a savage yank, pulling them right up between his cheeks.

He yelped and writhed against the friction. 'I'm sorry, miss,' he whimpered.

'No, you're not. But you will be.'

He shuddered and I peeled his underpants down, smacking his ass with my hand. There had to be some CP, but he was mainly a humiliation junkie. I made him stand in the middle of the room with his bare bottom on display while I paced around him, describing the punishments nasty little boys deserved. I threatened to cane him in front of the entire school. All the girls would point at him and giggle.

After a few minutes I slipped behind him and slowly slid his Calvins back up. He trembled with anticipation and then I yanked them up between his cheeks again. There was a satisfying rip of fabric.

'Oh dear,' I said. 'They seem to have torn. I'm afraid I don't have any replacements, but perhaps I can get you something from the girls' locker room. A pair of pink satin panties, maybe? I wonder what the other boys will say when they see you wearing those?'

He grew harder with every new humiliation I heaped on him.

A mirror covered one of the walls and I made him stand facing it with his hands on his head. Another wedgie and his expensive underpants tore again. When I told him it was a two-way mirror and that all the other boys were behind it, watching him, he turned to me, gasping and pleading with me to let him come. I smiled and told him no. His face crumpled in misery and I teased him for another ten minutes before I gave him permission to masturbate.

He dropped to his knees and made short work of it while I watched and then made him clean himself up with his torn underpants. I was beginning to understand the appeal of power and control.

'Wedgie Boy' became my most devoted regular client.

I'd played shrink many times when I was a stripper, but as a domme I got to do it for real. Gary was a fortysomething business executive who wanted to be the plaything of an unscrupulous woman. The problem was, he couldn't admit to himself that he had such fantasies. So he found a clever way to circumvent his guilt.

Ava had told me what he wanted because he didn't want to discuss it beforehand; he wanted me to be in character as soon as I entered the room. I was his therapist and he'd come to me for help with relieving the stress of his high-pressure job. But I was a sadistic bitch with wicked plans of my own. I suggested hypnosis.

I'd been hypnotised by a therapist once myself, so I stole some elements of what I remembered and made the session my own. I made him close his eyes and I guided his breathing. Long slow deep breaths. I had him descend a long staircase in his mind.

'Listen to my voice, Gary. Every step takes you deeper and deeper inside, deeper asleep. It's getting darker the further you go, but you can feel the steps. Down, down, down. You won't fall. My voice is guiding you. My voice is your whole world.'

Once he was under my spell I told him to strip. He obeyed instantly, as though in a trance. I ran him through a series of basic commands – sit, stand, raise your arms, stand on one leg. He never hesitated; he did everything I told him to do without a second's pause. He was so convincing that I worried I'd actually hypnotised him.

I saddled him and rode him round the room like a slow awkward pony, urging him on with a riding crop. I made him worship my feet. I had him bring me implements to beat him with. For an hour I had my way with him, giving him some marks to remember me by. Then it was time to snap him out of it.

'When I tell you to open your eyes you will remember nothing of the past hour. You won't even see the bruises. All you'll feel is a sense of relief and relaxation. Now – open your eyes.'

He blinked them open and smiled. I expected the game to be over and was about to ask him how it had been.

'You're right, Doctor,' he said. 'I do feel more relaxed. Thank you.'

I followed his lead and didn't break character. 'Er, good. Then I'll see you again next week, Mr Smith.'

I walked him to the door and instead of the customary hug I got a chaste handshake. 'Four o'clock on Tuesday,' he said, back in control.

When he left the room I felt oddly unsatisfied. Sure, it was his fantasy and he seemed content with it. But I was sad that he had to pretend the whole thing away afterwards. I told myself that if I saw him again I'd try to hypnotise him for real and plant the suggestion that it was OK to want such things. But he never came back.

34. AND HORROR THE SOUL OF THE PLOT

One day Ava said she had a special gig for me. 'None of the other girls will see this man. But I think you'll be fine with it.'

I was instantly on my guard. 'Why don't they want to see him?'

'They say he's too freaky. But he doesn't even want to do a scene – just talk to a "like-minded" person.'

'About what?'

She told me. Fascinated, I agreed to see him. But I had to do a bit of homework first.

Alfred was a small, frail man. He looked about seventy and his hands trembled as he talked. What little hair he had was white.

'I own a small island off the coast of South America,' he explained in a high reedy voice. 'I need you to help me run the compound.'

'Certainly,' I said, all business. I was dressed as if for a job interview. Sexy secretary with piled-up hair. Stockings and heels. 'I know a man who can organise the kidnapping and transport.'

He nodded approvingly at my interest and efficiency. 'I need at least ten girls. All between sixteen and eighteen. And slightly overweight.' He went on to describe the perfect skin type – pale, not olive.

Next he talked about the training compound and the fitness regime the girls would be subjected to. Again I knew someone who could oversee the operation and he discussed various nude exercises in detail with a dreamy expression. Naturally, the girls would be punished for any resistance.

'And when they're fit and ready . . .' He looked at me eagerly.

'Then we'll decide how to prepare and serve each one. I find that delicate sauces complement the meat best.' I smiled like a chef taking pride in her culinary skill as we discussed marinades, spices and seasoning. He licked his lips theatrically, embellishing my recipes with elaborate presentations. Silver chafing dishes. Liveried footmen. The works.

When I discussed the taste of human flesh, he clasped his hands delightedly. He nodded when I compared it to veal and I wondered fleetingly if he'd actually tasted girl cutlet. But perhaps he'd only read the account of William Buehler Seabrook, as I had. The *New York Times* reporter had famously cooked and eaten human meat, declaring that it tasted like 'good, fully developed veal'. All in the interest of research.

I enjoyed the gruesome fantasy scene, though I suspected any cannibal worth his salt would know that you don't slim girls down for slaughter; you fatten them up. Alfred told me afterwards that he'd had his first sexual response as a boy when his mother read him *Hansel and Gretel*. One boy's fairy tale is another boy's porn.

Niki plays the most believable brat and it would be hard to resist spanking her even if she was well behaved.

I have a feeling that many Englishmen would love to be able to spank American brats and it occurs to me that this might be a way to boost tourism to the UK. The tourism board could offer canings and spankings while staying in London and I am sure Virgin Airways could come up with a catchy ad campaign about flying their airline, featuring American girls with stripes on their bottoms. You never forget your first, um, caning that is.

From a review of *An American Brat in London*, produced by Strictly English

35. SCENES FROM A LIFE IN THE PAIN INDUSTRY

I'm naked. Strapped down over a rudimentary whipping frame, crying out as the woman to my left wields the cane without mercy. One stroke is followed by a terrific crack and then a soft clatter as the broken tip flies off and hits the wall. This doesn't stop my punisher. She simply flips the cane over and resumes. And when it breaks again she reaches into the bucket beside her for a fresh one.

When it's over Zbyšek yells 'Cut!' and I feel friendly hands undoing my bonds. Kateřina gathers up the broken cane fragments and shows them to me, giggling.

'Damn, Niki, what is your ass made of?' someone asks.

* * *

I've just taken my panties off. Suddenly, the changing-room door opens and a flock of elderly ladies comes in, chattering about their aerobics class. The small white-haired one in front looks at me and does a double-take at the sight of my shaved pussy. Most spanking models are bare, so it's easy to forget that it might be a shock to someone else. Especially at the gym at this early hour, where I'm the youngest female by twenty years.

I hurriedly turn away in embarrassment, remembering too late that the marks from my last shoot haven't faded. My cheeks are criss-crossed with vivid tramlines from Gillian Lancer's cane.

Flustered, I turn back around, inflicting the porn-shorn view on them as the lesser of evils while I dig behind me frantically for my towel.

The room is silent as I scurry off to the shower.

* * *

It's February, and 7 degrees Celsius. A misty rain is falling at Whitby Abbey on the chilly northeastern coast of England. People in heavy winter coats are exploring the ruins.

I climb up onto a broken column about six feet off the ground. Not naked. I'm in a black velvet formal evening gown and high heels. My shoulders and arms are bare and covered in gooseflesh. It's my first non-kinky modelling gig.

Balancing precariously on the crumbling stone, I strike a dramatic pose, trying not to look down. I raise my arms to hold my gauzy black wrap over my head so it flutters in the wind. A crowd starts to gather, watching with morbid fascination. Will she fall? Will she break her neck? How did the photographer get her to do that?

I climb down at last, stumbling as my heels sink into the muddy wet grass. Immensely relieved. I hadn't realised quite how high it was. I was shaking all over.

The photographer grins delightedly. 'You're game for anything, girl!'

I force myself to smile. If only I could be as fearless as my reputation.

* * *

My anxiety fades with every shot of *hruškovice*. David adjusts the headphones for me and the music starts again. I close my eyes, swaying to the soft leathery beat of the drums and the strumming of his acoustic guitar, leaning in close to the microphone. David's low husky voice winds through Leonard Cohen's words and I whisper along, a silky background echo.

Waiting . . . for the miracle . . .

I'm bolder by the next take and I can hardly even feel the cane marks from the *Stalin 2* shoot earlier that day. This is my first time in a recording studio and I've never sung with another person before. It's surprisingly intimate. Sexy. The pear brandy warms my throat, turning my breath into an erotic instrument. I'd protested that I wasn't a singer, but he said I didn't need to be.

'Just feel the music,' he said. 'Let it take you over. Let it possess you.'

Hands tied . . . hurt you . . . severe . . .

I surrender to the sex that is music as the words melt like snowflakes on my tongue.

Taken . . . begging . . . naked . . .

* * *

I'm naked. Secured by my wrists and ankles to the black St Andrew's cross in the prison basement while Officer Lewis sneers at me. Bradley is running her long nails up and down my punished flesh, making me gasp. I've been thrown to the wolves for trying to kill the prison governor with a pair of scissors.

Bradley yanks my hair and tells me in her thick Yorkshire accent that she'll enjoy making me suffer. And she does. The flogger is soft leather, but she lays on with a will. The pain is bearable, more like a massage than a whipping, but the psychological element does me in. They tell me that no one will care what happens to me down here, that I've really done it now and the rest of my sentence will be a living hell. They'll see to that.

The humiliation makes me weak and the focused attention makes me hot. The combination is devastatingly erotic. But it's that time of the month and my emotions are in turmoil. I've been on the verge of tears all day. All I need is a trigger.

I raise my head and suddenly my old delusion returns. Looking around the room, I imagine that my father is seeing it all through my eyes. The prison guards, the chains, the cameras, his little girl naked and whipped and turned on by it all . . . I close my eyes before he can see any more.

Again and again the leather tails lash my tender back. I'm afraid to open my eyes. Alone in the darkness with my pain and my shameful arousal, I can't banish the spectre of my father. I'm terrified he'll find out what I do, that he'll hate me. I'll be the family's filthy secret. I've never confronted the fear in such a vulnerable state before. Time seems to slow down as I imagine the emotional annihilation. I'm falling. The ground is rushing up to meet me fast. This is it – my worst fear.

As the terror starts to consume me I remember where I am and what I'm doing here. The pain brings me back to myself and I feel strengthened by it. Comforted, as though by an old friend. This is me. This is who I am.

The show must go on. *Use it.*

I push the panic aside, transforming the despair into catharsis and giving in to my tears. It tastes like freedom. I'm still purging the angst when Leia yells 'Cut!'

Lewis drops his stern guard persona to comfort me and Leia walks unsteadily out from behind the camera, wiping her eyes. 'Dear God,' she says, her voice quavering. 'I just couldn't take any more.'

'I'm fine,' I reassure her, instantly back to normal and stunned by her distress. 'Hey, it's OK. I'm the one who got beaten, after all!' The demons have been exorcised and I'm free once more.

Leia forces a smile. 'Sorry. That was just . . . intense. Empathy, you know?'

Oh, yes. I know.

* * *

'It's a little bit cold,' Ben says without a trace of sympathy.

Wolfgang opens the door to show me where we'll be shooting this time. The numbing chill penetrates me as I take in my surroundings. I've stepped straight into a horror film.

Long metal countertops line the frigid room. On a rack above my head, sharp meat hooks clink together, glinting in the harsh light. Butcher knives and saws hang like threats on the walls around me.

I approach the steel table in the centre of the room with trepidation. I'm already shivering from the cold, even in my robe. I touch the sterile surface and wince at the chill. It's like ice. My handprint fades like the stain of warm breath from a mirror.

'I'm going to be lying naked on that?' I gulp.

'Of course!' Ben says.

Wolfgang raises a heavy meat cleaver and grins at me maniacally.

I love these guys.

Wow, your new movie *The Spy* looks hot! I haven't even finished my coffee, but I'm awake now!

Niki, you have got to be one of the best video 'victims' out there because you're not afraid to take pain, plus, it's OBVIOUS you're in pain and you react so well to it! (Some films, either they're winking at the camera or they look like they've been drugged, or they barely react at all.) Not to mention that your punishments always seem more real because you don't go willingly . . . and your face is extremely expressive. Also . . . I liked the face slapping shot . . .

So I'm a sick b*tch, what can I tell you?

Brooklyn Babe, New York

36. DON'T MENTION THE WAR

'*Ich bin kein Spion!*'

Sturmbannführer Feldmann doesn't believe me. His superiors have told him I'm a spy. And down here in the straw-filled basement, it's his word against mine.

I'm tied down on a bench, pleading with him to stop as he brings the razor strop down on my bottom again and again. My back still bears marks from the whipping he strung me up for earlier.

He asks me again who I'm working for.

'Deutschland!' I insist.

Another stroke. I howl with pain, begging him to let me go. '*Bitte, mein Herr, lass mich gehen!*'

I don't have the vocabulary to defend myself with more sophistication than that and I don't dare retreat into English. That would only make him more likely to see me as an English spy.

When I refuse to talk he unties me and I cower in the straw.

'*Morgen,*' he warns. '*Ich werde zurückkommen.*' Tomorrow he'll be back.

It was one of my German fans who wrote to Peter Schober at pain4fem, asking him to shoot a military interrogation scene with me.

'I hope you will resist,' he said on my blog. 'Let Peter know he cannot break you with his soft lashes!'

I'd enjoyed Peter's work in several movies and was eager to work with him. Pain4fem clearly took a lot of pride in their productions and there was a real attempt at storytelling. They were also fond of back whipping, which I found exciting and which my fans wanted to see. An interrogation with Peter (in German!) sounded right up my street.

An Austrian-Slovakian joint venture, pain4fem was located in Bratislava, forty miles east of Vienna. They were another unknown quantity in the Western world. Once again I would play intrepid explorer.

'Bratislava?' My friend Adam gasped. 'But that's where *Hostel* takes place!'

I had no idea what to expect. I was going by myself and Peter would meet me at the airport. He and his wife Helen had both been very friendly in email. When I asked about accommodation, Peter said I would be staying in their house and eating at their table; I was their guest.

'That's exactly what *I'd* say if I wanted to torture and kill a girl.'

Adam was right. In a way.

It's scary getting on a plane alone and turning up in a foreign country to be met by strangers. But it's all part of the head trip. Meeting new people is stressful for me, but by now my habit of being violently ill before every shoot was diminishing.

Peter is imposingly tall, so I spotted him right away. The cameraman, Jozo, was there too. As usual, everyone's English was better than my German, so we all chatted in English on the way to the studio.

I knew that pain4fem had never worked with a Western girl, but I was surprised to learn that they'd never shot with a professional spanking model at all. Most of the models they hired were vanilla Czech girls, probably from the same model pool Lupus dipped into. There was no BDSM scene in the area and no way to find enthusiasts.

Peter's a genuinely kinky guy who'd fantasised about spanking all his life. But the reality of causing actual pain to girls had turned out to be less fun than he'd imagined. I found his non-sadism endearing and I marvelled that he could be so stern and ruthless on camera.

'So what's the story for the movie?' I asked.

'It will be a military interrogation, like your German friend wrote. It's the 1940s and you're accused of being an English spy. I'll play a Nazi.'

When he saw my stunned expression he laughed, misunderstanding. 'Don't be worried. You are safe with us.'

I wasn't worried; I was thinking about *The Night Porter*. Nazis
as a sexual fantasy: the ultimate villains, the ultimate taboo. I felt
the instant combination of arousal and guilt that that most potent
of images always triggers in me.

I flashed back to the previous October. Skin Two's Rubber Ball
in London. The vaulted arches beneath London Bridge Station
house the city's largest nightclub. That night the 30,000-square-
foot venue was teeming with people in the most outrageous outfits
imaginable. Everything from Elizabethan court dress to latex
mummification suits. It was my first fetish ball and it was an
unforgettable experience in more ways than one.

Nazi chic is banned from most UK fetish events, but the Rubber
Ball is an exception. I was there with Lee and Sergei and at one
point we got separated. Lost in the labyrinth and getting
increasingly anxious, I battled my way through the crowds
trying to find them again. Suddenly I turned a corner and found
myself face to face with a man in full authentic SS uniform.
Swastikas and all. The sight left me breathless and I stood staring
wide-eyed until I recovered enough to move aside and let him
pass.

I couldn't process my feelings. I was shocked, frightened,
horrified, excited, ashamed. Fascinated. My face flushed, my heart
pounding, I tried to resist the masochistic fantasies that invaded
my mind. I was a captured Resistance fighter, interrogated by the
SS. The daughter of a German officer accused of treason, made to
suffer in his place. A girl who simply wanted a comfortable war
and earned it by sleeping with the enemy.

Sylvia Plath's black observation isn't entirely ironic: 'Every
woman adores a Fascist.'

Peter outlined a story that fully explored my dark side.

Mary is an English girl working as a translator for the Germans.
She falls under suspicion and it's Peter's job to make her admit to
being a spy. He does all manner of coercive things to her down in
the basement, but she refuses to confess. Even after a severe back
whipping, strapping and caning. When he realises he'll get
nothing from her, he decides to have some fun. He'd joked earlier
about getting into Mary's pants, so while she's still tied down on
the table, he claims his prize.

Cut to Helen upstairs, listening in amusement to the sounds from below. 'That horny old goat.' She chuckles.

In the basement, Peter's doing up his trousers, telling Mary there's no further use for her. He pulls out a gun.

Cut back to Helen, on the phone. Her superior informs her that there's been a mistake: Mary's not a British spy after all.

BANG!

'Oops ... I'm afraid you're too late,' she says with a shrug. 'Better send us a new translator.'

I particularly liked the wicked guilt-free denouement. I had never imagined *I'd* be playing a Nazi! The story was controversial, but so was my whole career. I was gradually working my way through history's most infamous tyrants: the StB, the Stasi and now the Nazis. I'd come a long way from my adolescent days of agonising over my uncomfortable fantasies; now I was living them. Every single one of them.

It was an impressive set-up. The studio occupied the entire multi-room basement of a large house. It was crammed with props and costumes and lighting equipment. And yet the whole crew only consisted of Peter, Helen and Jozo. All three worked the cameras, but Peter was writer, director, actor, cameraman and editor. He also built all the punishment apparatus.

People joke about amateur films being shot by a couple of guys in a basement. Well, that was exactly the set-up here, but pain4fem's movies were anything but amateur. I was amazed that such high-quality productions could come from such a skeleton crew.

Pain4fem also had an interesting payment scale. Instead of a flat fee for my time or for the film itself, they paid by the stroke. We would spend the first day shooting short clips for their website. I would get a nominal fee for those, but the majority of the payment would be for the caning and whipping in the film. The rate was €10 per stroke for 'hard' strokes and €20 for 'very hard' strokes.

'It's all up to you,' Peter said. 'During the shoot we will take short breaks and you decide how many strokes and how hard. And if anything is too much for you, the safeword is *jablako*. It means "apple" in Slovak.'

It wasn't like Lupus, where you signed on for the ride and it was all or nothing. I had complete control this time, which was reassuring.

The clips were fun, but not very strenuous. As usual, they weren't heavy on plot or dialogue. I didn't have to say much beyond '*Nein! Bitte!*' We did a couple of schoolgirl scenes, a mediaeval back whipping and a judicial strapping. There was also a foot caning for their bastinado website.

For each scene, Peter would give me one stroke of whichever implement he was using – strap, paddle, flogger – and then cut to ask if I was OK. After that we'd do five strokes at a time until we reached a reasonable total, shooting stills in between the action scenes. That way the stills would show a sensible build-up of marks. Then we'd break for an hour so the redness could fade and we could shoot the next clip with my bottom pristine and unmarked. After every scene Peter would grin sheepishly and say 'Sorry' in a meek little voice.

I only used the safeword once. In the judicial strapping, Peter moved from my bottom to the backs of my thighs. First one stroke. Then another. My thighs are out of bounds, but I'd neglected to tell him that. I didn't want to ruin the shot by safewording, so I figured I'd just wait for the next break and tell him then. But after the third stroke I wimped out.

I waited a few seconds to allow room for editing to cover the break. '*Jablako!*'

Instantly Peter was beside me. 'Are you OK? Is it too hard?'

I explained the problem and he apologised profusely.

'No, no,' I reassured him. 'It's my fault. I should have told you.'

But he seemed genuinely upset that he'd hurt me. I tried to convince him it wasn't a big deal. The redness would certainly fade in an hour.

'Will you be all right? We can stop there if you want.'

'I'm fine, really,' I said with a laugh, embarrassed by the fuss he was making. It's funny how often the bottom is the one having to reassure the top. Eventually I persuaded him to continue and we finished the scene. Then it was time for lunch.

By the time we got to the last clip of the day, we'd run out of implements. Peter looked around the toy cupboard and found a carpet beater.

'Works for me,' I said.

The cameras rolled. Peter came home and caught me reading a magazine when I was supposed to be studying. He yelled something at me in German and I had to pretend I understood. I guessed that he was threatening to spank me. Sure enough, he grabbed the carpet beater and made me bend over the sofa. I was wearing my favourite pair of hot pants with 'criminal' written across the cheeks in a grungy font. He commented on them disapprovingly before giving me the first whack.

'Cut! Are you OK, Niki?'

'Yeah, I'm fine.' The stop-start pace was exhausting.

We started again and he took the hot pants down, continuing on the bare. It stung more than I expected it to and I yelped and kicked, just as I had all day. The scenes were starting to blend into one another and I was looking forward to the film.

At last the final clip was done and Peter offered his familiar half-hearted apology for treating me so horribly. I couldn't help but wonder how the vanilla models reacted.

I was tired of doing clips and my bottom was feeling tender, but I was also disappointed that I hadn't had an over-the-knee spanking in my pyjamas. They're the classic style with long sleeves – white flannel with girlish pink hearts. It's a favourite scene for both tops and bottoms. There's just something so intimate and comforting about a bedtime smacking in your PJs.

Peter saw them as I was repacking my suitcase and he read my mind. 'I'm sorry,' he said, grinning, 'but you will have to make one more scene with me.'

I grinned back, squirming.

That evening, we had to shoot all the set-up shots and non-CP scenes for the movie. Peter and Helen got dressed and I was relieved to see that they weren't using actual Nazi regalia. They wore armbands with a made-up symbol. The uniforms themselves were khaki and wouldn't pass muster with any historical re-enactment society, but they would work as a fantasy. It was good enough for me.

Peter said he'd have to concentrate on speaking proper high German instead of his slangy Austrian dialect. I hadn't known there was a difference, but hearing him make the shift was enlightening. 'Hochdeutsch' is the German equivalent of BBC English. Truly the language of authority.

He'd printed out a list of German military ranks and made himself the equivalent of a major, with Helen subordinate to him. He wrote the names on the printout and set it aside. He was having a ball clowning around in the uniform, hamming it up and barking at Helen to help him put on his boots. She bore it all with an indulgent smile.

In the first scene, *Sturmbannführer* Feldmann and Fräulein Rettich are complaining about the lousy wartime coffee in the French château they've commandeered. Feldmann rants about the imminent glory of world domination when Mary arrives with some translated files. She shyly bids them good night, going upstairs to bed. Feldmann watches her go, a lecherous twinkle in his eye. 'She'll soon warm up to me,' he says. 'I'll have her.' Then the phone rings and it's his superior. They've got information on the suspected spy: it's Mary!

Simple enough.

We did my bit with the files. (I couldn't pronounce the German word, so we made it 'papers' instead.) Peter watched me go and muttered about me to Helen. He strode to the table with the convincing 1940s-era phone and the not-so-convincing 2000-era map of Slovakia (not actually a separate country in World War II). He picked up the receiver and faltered.

'I forgot my name.'

After consulting the printout we started again. But this time when he got to the phone he noticed that his armband was falling off. Helen stapled it to his sleeve and we started again.

Peter marched over to the phone and picked it up. '*Jawohl!*' he said sharply. '*Sturmbannführer . . . Scheisse!* What's my name?'

'Feldmann!' we all chorused.

Back to the phone. '*Sturmbannführer Feldmann hier.*' He continued on in German, asking what information they had on this spy. He listened, frowned and agreed that he would get the truth out of Mary. 'OK,' he said at last and hung up. Then he paused, catching himself. ' "OK"? "OK" is American! I speak German!'

After we stopped laughing, Jozo offered, '*Jawohl!*'

'And "Feldmann"!' I reminded him.

This time he made it through the phone call, but he was playing it up so much by this point that Helen developed an incurable case of the giggles. It took all her willpower not to crack up through the next round of takes.

Finally, they made it to the end of the scene. Feldmann took a gun out of the drawer and they went upstairs to haul poor Mary out of bed in her nightgown. Helen kept the gun pointed at me while Peter dragged me down the stairs and I asked frantically what I'd done.

Two hours later, we were finished. In the final cut, this whole scene takes all of five minutes. I couldn't wait to see the gag reel.

37. THE SPY

I love resistance play, especially with someone I have no hope of besting. Peter's a big guy, so I could struggle as hard as I liked.

Down in the cellar, he sat me down hard in a chair and tied my hands behind my back with a coarse length of hemp rope. He asked who I was working for and when he didn't like my answer he slapped me across the face. (We'd negotiated €10 for that.) I insisted that I didn't know what he was talking about. He brandished the gun at me and I flinched away, flashing back to *Stalin 2* and Brandon Lee.

When we stopped Peter asked if I was OK. I assured him I was. I found the interrogation scenario highly erotic and I didn't want to have to keep stopping like we had for the clips the day before. I just wanted to lose myself in the fantasy. It was strange for me, doing a whole movie in such short bursts. I didn't really have time to get into the headspace. And once he yelled 'Cut', Peter was totally out of character, joking and horsing around with Helen, whom he wouldn't stop calling 'Fräulein Rettich'.

As soon as he called 'Action!' he was my evil interrogator again, shifting seamlessly between brutality and boyish enthusiasm at playing the bad guy. It wasn't so easy for me. I couldn't go instantly from camp to terror. Clearly there would be no Method acting here.

It was time for the back whipping. Peter secured my bound wrists to a chain above my head and asked how many strokes I could take. 'I don't know,' I said, not knowing how painful it would be. 'Let's see how it goes.'

'Five strokes at a time?'

'Sure.'

Back whipping is something I've always found extremely hot. I had fantasised about it often, but I hadn't actually experienced it much. Cameron had flogged me a few times in roleplay scenes. And Sergei often liked to whip my back and my feet (usually because I had either just done a shoot or had one coming up and my bottom was off-limits). At the Rubber Ball he'd tied me to an X-shaped grating in the centre of the room and painted some pretty stripes on my back with a four-foot singletail. But this was to be my first *severe* back whipping. Exactly what the more sadistic members of my Yahoo group had been clamouring for.

Any spanko will tell you that a bottom is made for smacking. It's well padded. A back has no such luxury. A whipping on the back stings terribly, though it doesn't cause the deep bruising you can get from heavier implements designed for the bottom.

Peter drew back the braided leather whip and cracked it across my upper back again and again. I cried out, writhing in pain and begging for mercy in broken German. The pain was intense and this time I could I let go, abandoning myself to it.

He lashed me mercilessly, asking me why I wouldn't talk. He teased me with the whip, playing it over my breasts. The language, the scenario, the sensations . . . I was overwhelmed. Electric currents raced through my body, pushing me to that strange secret place where pain shades into pleasure.

I was disoriented whenever Peter cut to check on me and do stills. Every interruption was like being doused with cold water. *Forget the movie*, I was tempted to say. *Let's just do the roleplay!*

Occasionally Peter would pause after a stroke to ask me another bullying question, but I didn't always understand what he was saying. The character may have been a translator, but the actress wasn't so fluent. All I could offer was 'I'm not a spy!' I was kicking myself afterwards for not having the presence of mind to say, 'Surely a spy would speak better German!'

He gave me twenty strokes in total, but I refused to confess, insisting that I was on *their* side. Peter made the last five count and I broke down in tears, incapable of pleading, but thrilled at the emotional release. Pain never provokes tears the way that psychological triggers do. I savoured the rush, surfed the pain.

Feldmann untied me and I collapsed in the straw. He told me to think about what I wanted to say before he returned the next day. Then he stalked out, leaving me to comfort myself. He kicked straw over me, but I hardly noticed. I was floating somewhere on the other side of the pain. I was gone. The cameras ran and I sat there crying, in misery, in ecstasy. Devastated.

When I finally drifted back to earth, Peter offered me his usual rueful grin. 'Sorry. I hope you don't hate me too much for that.'

I managed a smile through my tears. *What's to hate?* I thought.

Jozo took some stills and I looked over my shoulder at the monitors, amazed and delighted to see the vivid scarlet stripes. The diagonal welts ran from the top of my right shoulder to the bottom of my left shoulder blade. A left-handed flogger could have crossed all the X's with dramatic effect. There's something artistic – elegant, even – about a back that's been well whipped.

All of a sudden, the front doorbell rang. Peter and Helen looked at each other and then down at their uniforms. Helen waved the gun and mimed throwing open the door to shoot the intruder. Finally, they shrugged and marched upstairs to see who it was. I stared after them in amazement. Maybe it's nothing unusual in Bratislava for people to answer the door wearing Nazi uniforms.

Once they'd got rid of the visitor, the torment resumed. Feldmann and Rettich returned to find their prisoner curled up asleep on the bench, clutching her torn nightgown for meagre cover. Peter planted his boot against my rear, shoving me off the bench and tumbling me into the straw. That part was my idea; I am a stuntgirl, after all.

We broke for lunch and then it was time for the caning. Neither the whip nor the razor strop had broken me. This was my final chance. They tied me down spread-eagled over a battered table and I trembled, my skin prickling with cold sweat. The rough edge of the table bit sharply into my stomach, but I knew that would soon be the least of my worries.

I expected it to be severe and Peter didn't disappoint. My bottom was already raw and sore from the razor strop, not to mention the previous day's shooting. After the first five strokes, Peter asked how many I wanted. I suggested thirty.

'Hard or very hard?'

Well, 'hard' was painful enough, so I decided to stay at that level for now and then make the last five count. It would be the perfect finale.

And *mein Gott*, did they count!

I was sobbing before it was over, on another intense high. But I felt oddly disconnected from my emotions. I usually empathise with what my character is suffering – even Čermaková, the gangster's daughter. But this time I was as much a villain as my tormentor. No one had to feel guilty about Mary's treatment, however unfair. She was a filthy traitor, a Nazi sympathiser who was getting what she deserved.

I wanted her to suffer. Instead of feeling sorry for her, I revelled in her pain and anguish. And yet she was *me*. It wasn't masochism; it was self-sadism. And it translated sexually. I wanted to be cheapened, humiliated, degraded. The shame was rapturous. I cried for a long time after the cameras stopped, deliriously aroused. I had reached a deep submissive zone and lost all sense of reality. It was like succumbing to some bizarre kind of sexual madness. I didn't want to be sane again.

I was also grieving for the end of the scene. I knew I'd had enough, but I still *hadn't had enough*. You get greedy when the euphoria starts to fade. It's a drug you don't ever want to wear off. But it can't last forever.

I had one last little scene, though it didn't involve any pain.

The night before, I had sent gleeful text messages to Cameron and Sergei about the scenario. 'My second rape scene,' I gushed. 'And my first death!'

This was it. My big moment.

Peter tried to describe what he wanted. 'I don't know how to say it in English, but when I ... um ... enter you ... But not really! Faked! When I ... well ...'

'Don't worry. I know what to do.' I said it with all the confidence of a seasoned prostitute reassuring a nervous customer.

The camera zooms in on a pair of boots and breeches behind Mary's bare legs. The trousers fall, covering the boots. Cut to Mary's horrified face. She cries out rhythmically and the camera pans back to the boots as their wearer thrusts against the table again and again. It looks intense on film, but it's so hard to take these scenes seriously when you're shooting them. I suspect actual sex would be easier to film; the coyness makes it all a bit silly and self-conscious. Especially when your rapist's wife is the one behind the camera!

I had to stay in position while they filmed Peter fastening his trousers and preparing to shoot me. The rest was all sound effects:

Chopin's 'Funeral March' and a gunshot heard off-screen as Rettich gets the news over the phone. And the reassuring text afterwards: 'Don't worry; it's only a movie.' So very Peter.

The funny thing is, I had anticipated a very dark and brutal shooting experience, given the subject matter. Something like *Stalin 3*. But the overall mood was light-hearted and frivolous, with so much goofing off between takes that I couldn't disappear into the fantasy. I imagined the outtakes would be longer than the film. It didn't occur to me until some time afterwards that the actual film would bear little resemblance to my memory of shooting it. Thank God for DVD extras.

Niki,

It always amazes me how you girls willingly submit or allow them to tie you down. I think they would have to drag me kicking and screaming, especially knowing what is coming. I can appreciate how the anticipation, dread and fear of the pain can be a very powerful and stimulating thing. The high and glow you get afterwards must be worth it.

Don't know how you do it. There must be a point where you feel you can't take any more, yet the punishment goes on. Can't say it looks like you enjoy your work, but you must.

Cane and Ginger, UK

38. THE LONGEST TWO MINUTES OF MY LIFE

M ost big cities have a BDSM scene if you know where to look. The organised groups fly under the radar with oblique names like Posterity Club, Crimson Moon and Florida Moonshine.

Based in Tampa, Florida Moonshine is run by two expat Brits, Tony Hamilton and Ian Head (a.k.a. The London Tanner). When Shadow Lane decided not to have a Valentine's Day party one year, Tony and Ian organised one of their own. Cameron and I had lots of friends who were planning to go, Bailey among them. We were both looking forward to seeing her again. We also arranged to spend a few days in the Everglades after the party.I love travelling and seeing new places. I love road trips and boats and trains. But I absolutely hate flying.

Different things scare different people. Pain scares me and I often have sleepless nights before severe shoots. But it's the devil I know. It's a fear I'm compelled to confront, a fear I've come to love. I feel empowered every time I conquer it, like I've charmed a deadly snake. And no matter how scary or non-consensual it looks on film, in reality I always have control; I can make it stop. Flying is different. On an airplane I have no control at all.

Somewhere over the Atlantic, the pilot warned us that we'd be hitting some turbulence. I dread hearing that. But I always watch the flight attendants and they never look bothered, no matter how bumpy it gets. It keeps me calm and I trust that they'd know if something was truly wrong. But when the plane starts yawing so violently the pilot tells them to be seated, I get worried. And when it drops several hundred feet without warning, I panic.

This was the worst turbulence I'd ever experienced. The fifteen minutes we were threatened with stretched into an hour and a half of learning what clothes feel like in the tumble dryer. My stomach plummeted with every sharp dive the plane made and my heartbeat was deafening in my ears. A barrage of images assaulted me: a wing tearing free of the plane, the roof peeling open with a metallic shriek, passengers sucked out into the storm . . .

When I found myself thinking, *Please let it be quick*, I started to cry.

'But you love roller coasters,' Cameron said, surprised by the extremity of my reaction.

'Roller coasters don't crash into the ocean,' I blubbered. 'They run on tracks and they don't come off them.'

I knew intellectually that I was safe. I knew that. So, while I was clutching Cameron's arm and squealing at every sudden lurch, I was also painfully aware of how irrationally I was behaving. But fear is irrational; it bypasses all your reasoning. I can't control the panic any more than I can control the plane. It was truly awful to look around and see other passengers asleep or reading peacefully while I was holding on to Cameron in tears, utterly certain that we were all about to die. As with pain, it's not death that scares me; it's the *dying*.

I wish I could find a way to eroticise my fear of flying. If you have any ideas, please let me know.

After a five-hour delay in Amsterdam, a terrible flight and a missed connection, we found ourselves stuck overnight in Detroit. In February. In Florida clothes. I'm a desert girl and I'm not good with cold. The airline arranged a shuttle to a nearby hotel, but we nearly froze waiting for it in the snow. They gave us dinner vouchers, but the restaurant was closed by the time we got to the hotel they sent us to, so we had pie and fruit juice from a kiosk for dinner. At 2 a.m. To top it off, Cameron had picked up an eye infection. We could only hope there'd be a kinky doctor at the party who could prescribe something for it.

Our spirits lifted when we finally made it to Tampa. At last we could see our friends and put the travelling fiasco behind us, though we worried that disasters were becoming the rule rather than the exception. On our previous transatlantic flight, Continental had lost our luggage for 72 hours, promising to reimburse us for 'essentials' we had to buy in the meantime. I went straight to Victoria's Secret and blew my $100 allotment on panties. Hey, you need clean underwear every day.

At least this time our toys and costumes had arrived with us. And the unexpected night in Detroit didn't affect the party; we'd left two days early to have time to recover from the jet-lag.

Ian picked us up from the airport and took us out to his place in the country – 'the world headquarters of the London Tanners', as he called it. It was great to see Bailey again and we immediately started scheming about scenes to play. Cameron and Tony had arranged to give a caning demo and they'd volunteered Bailey and me. We wore matching Japanese school uniforms and slipped away into the adjoining room to psych ourselves up when we saw how big the audience was. There were about fifty people crammed into the suite – all there to see us caned.

Eventually Cameron found us and dragged us out by our ears. We stood not-so-quietly to the side while the men gave a short history of canes and caning in English schools. Technique. Safety.

'Yeah, yeah, blah blah blah,' we said, pushing and scuffling in our corner.

Cameron separated us while Tony displayed various types of canes to the audience.

Bailey yanked my hair and I cried out loudly.

Tony gave us a warning look. 'I think it might be time for a practical demonstration,' he said. 'Come here.'

It was performance time. Up went the pleated skirts, down came the white cotton knickers, and SWISH! went the cane across our bottoms. We played to the crowd, making cheeky comments and yelping dramatically when the strokes landed.

I loved being objectified like that. Having my bottom exposed for such a businesslike demonstration made me very hot. No matter how bratty we were, the men stayed impartial and detached. I felt like a research subject in a scientific experiment. I imagined I didn't even have a name, just a number. I squirmed each time I felt Tony's cane, listening to his soft upper-crust accent as he demonstrated how to position the implement for maximum effect. Next to me, Cameron was being equally impartial with Bailey, discussing the efficacy of waiting between strokes to allow the sting to build and subside.

The highlight of the demo was the 'horsing' display. It's a traditional position you rarely get to see in movies and one I'd always wanted to try in a scene. Bailey stood behind me and I bent my knees so she could put her arms over my shoulders. I took her wrists and hoisted her up on my back, bending forward and raising her up well off the floor for Cameron's cane.

I'd been next to other girls when they were caned before. I'd been face to face with them too. But I'd never had another girl on my back while she was caned. The audience loved it and I wish I could have seen it. I don't really want to be horsed myself, but I enjoyed holding Bailey in place. Even if she did scream in my ear.

She saved Cameron, though. Sometime after the demo she overheard a fragment of conversation. Someone had mentioned being a doctor.

She pounced on him. 'You're a doctor? In that case I have a terribly rude question for you.'

He was kind enough to look at Cameron's eye and write him a prescription. And another kind soul offered to drive him to a pharmacy, as neither of us knew the area. Though neither of them expected anything in return, I wouldn't let their altruism to go unrewarded. I offered myself to both men in turn – my bottom, anyway. I enjoyed the play immensely, but I like to think of it as payment for services rendered. Ah, if only it worked like that in the real world.

Bailey has a lot of fans, but none as devoted as Jeoffry. He was a regular on a spanking forum she and I both posted on and he'd come to the party specifically to meet her. We were both flattered when he asked us to sign his DVD of *The Conspiracy*.

In one forum post Bailey had described a heavy tawse Ian had made for Cameron as a gift when she was visiting us. Ian said it was the best leather he'd ever seen, very much like that used in the genuine Lochgelly tawses of the past. He knew Cameron would appreciate it and he liked the idea of that special implement being used on Bailey and me. As with most of Ian's toys, we hated the vicious thing, along with the farmer who'd cultivated such thick cows.

At the end of the party, Jeoffry said he had a gift for Bailey. After reading her account of the nasty tawse, he'd written to Ian to commission one just like it. And here it was.

I wish I could have seen the 'Gee, thanks' expression on her face. It certainly made Jeoffry happy. And I think Bailey was secretly pleased as well, though she wasn't in a hurry to feel its sting.

Sadly, Jeoffry missed our impromptu performance at the vendor's fair. I don't know quite how it began, but somehow we started trading insults. I shoved her and she shoved back. I had an armload of freebies I'd been gathering and I threw them to the floor. Heads turned. Bailey took a step closer and we faced off like gunfighters, each waiting for the other to make the first move.

Suddenly we were locked in struggle, pulling hair and tearing at clothes. I dragged Bailey to the floor, where I straddled her and pinned her down. She responded by trying to bite my arm. A circle of people formed around us like spectators at a schoolyard scrap, cheering us on. Everyone loves a catfight and we were playing to the crowd. Bailey threw her leg over me and rolled me onto my back, where she tried to pin me down. I was stronger and I managed to escape, grabbing her long hair.

She turned the tables soon enough and I found myself on my back again, my strength waning. I knew I was the bad guy, so I was prepared to give in and let Bailey win. So I kicked feebly as she held my arms down on the floor and I surrendered. The crowd applauded and suddenly I was self-conscious. I hadn't intended to put on a show; I'd just felt like horsing around with Bailey.

Unfortunately, horsing around with Bailey would soon lead to one of the most embarrassing moments of my entire kink life.

About 25 of us made a dinner reservation at a nearby steakhouse that night. After the promised ten-minute wait had stretched into an hour, the staff finally seated us at a long table against the wall. Cameron and I sat furthest in, all the way in the corner. Bailey sat across from me.

Appetisers arrived to compensate us for our wait. By that time we were ravenous, so we dug into the bread and fried onions. The waiter was a friendly young Hispanic guy with a nice sense of humour. We weren't being terribly discreet about our conversation and he made a comment about the waitress being the one who administered spankings.

'Can I lick that off, Niki?'

I glanced down at my shirt. Bailey was pointing to the dip I'd spilled directly on my left breast.

I grinned. 'I don't think the waiter would mind.'

She leaned across the table and dragged her tongue across the spill, porn star-style while Cameron made a disapproving face. The waiter beamed.

'Thanks, Bailey,' I said.

We ordered dinner and Bailey and I jousted with our steak knives. We were wired from the weekend and disappointed that it was drawing to a close. I was in can't-get-enough mode.

'If you can't behave,' Cameron said. 'You're going over my knee.'

'Yeah, right,' I scoffed. 'In the middle of a crowded restaurant.'

A restaurant crowded with spankos, I should have reminded myself. And that included the waiter.

In an attempt to have the last word I plunged my knife down into my filet mignon, making a startlingly loud noise. I thought I'd broken the plate. The restaurant went silent.

'Right,' said Cameron. 'That does it.' He hauled me out of my chair and over his lap.

'No! Not here!' I was mortified. Even though most of the table had seen me spanked and caned all weekend, this was different. The venue changed everything.

Cameron gave me a few sharp swats over my camo trousers. I don't know how loud it was in reality, but I was so embarrassed I imagined the whole restaurant could hear it. I glared at him when he let me back up, petulantly rubbing my bottom.

'And now, young lady, you can stand in the corner.'

I turned scarlet. A few harmless smacks I could handle. I could laugh that off. Not the humiliation of cornertime – in public!

'My steak will get cold,' I offered in desperation.

'Your steak's already cold; it's half raw.'

'But . . . But . . .'

'All right. You can finish your dinner, but then you're going in the corner. For two minutes.'

That may not sound like much, but, believe me, it's an eternity, even in private. I ate as slowly as I could, praying it was all a bluff. It wasn't.

I tried to be brave. With a sigh I started to unfasten my trousers, as though he'd intended for me to stand in the corner bare-bottomed. Perhaps I could horrify him into changing his mind. Or at least convince him it wouldn't faze me. I'd pay for it later, of course. But not in the steakhouse.

Cameron called my bluff. 'Leave your trousers where they are and get in the corner. Hands on your head.'

The waiter appeared just as I obeyed and I made a final attempt to embarrass Cameron into sparing me.

'Oh, sir, not the paddle!' I said loudly, encouraged by the laughter at the table.

Cameron just gave me another swat and turned me around to face the corner. 'Two minutes.'

I squirmed and writhed in the corner, my face scorched with embarrassment. Everyone was watching. All the spankos at our table and all the vanilla diners in the restaurant. I could feel their eyes boring into me. Cornertime is bad enough one-on-one, but it's much worse with others watching. I'd been subjected to it in front of kinky friends or in scenes with one or two other players. *Never* in public. I imagined parents whispering to their children: 'See? You're never too old . . .' The only comfort was knowing they couldn't see my face. I didn't dare try to make light of it now.

It's only two minutes, I told myself. Counting the seconds in my head would make it last forever, but it was impossible not to focus on the time. I convinced myself I could hear every watch in the room ticking slowly, loudly, counting off the moments of my humiliation with excruciating deliberation.

To my horror, I realised the waiter hadn't left. He was standing right there, watching. 'We've got a dunce cap in the back,' he told Cameron casually. 'In case you need it.'

It was the longest two minutes of my life. When I was finally allowed to rejoin the table, I couldn't look at anyone. My face felt sunburned from blushing. Bailey gave me a guilty little smile; she'd been spared. Later, back in the same suite where we'd held the caning demo that morning, she held my hands and whispered encouragement while Cameron strapped my bare bottom with Ian's gift. Everyone who'd been at our table sat watching like the board of governors at a reformatory. Tony even took pictures.

It was one of those deliriously ambiguous situations – utterly mortifying and yet intensely erotic. Perhaps even *more* erotic for the humiliation. What had been almost unbearable in the restaurant was made sexual by the change of venue. And what had been hot about the businesslike caning demo was made edgy by the situation – a public punishment. I was torn between hating it and loving it.

'It's almost over,' Bailey whispered, giving my hands a sisterly squeeze as the final six strokes made me yelp and kick.

I recalled my first thought of her on the road trip to Denver: *I hope I like this Bailey girl.*

I definitely did.

Hi Niki,

I'm unsure if you'll ever read this as I've just seen some quite upsetting pictures. The first 2 show you next to a fearsome alligator. But in the third there is only a contented-looking gator with a Niki-shaped bulge in its stomach.

A world without Niki would be very dull indeed and I just hope the bulge was coincidental and not the upsetting demise of Miss Flynn.

Lots of love, hugs and swats,

Erik, Glasgow

39. WHAT BIG TEETH YOU HAVE . . .

Sore-bottomed and bruised, Bailey and I said goodbye.
Cameron and I left the party and headed south, to the
Everglades. It's a place of strange and striking beauty. Swollen
cypress trees rise from the swamp, trailing clumps of Spanish moss
in the murky water. Shy manatees swim in the mangrove forests
that form the Barrier Islands. Giant wading birds stand majesti-
cally in the shallows. And scattered along the banks – absolutely
everywhere – are alligators.

I'd seen them in zoos, but never in the wild. They're fascinating
creatures and I couldn't take enough pictures of them. I felt like
a little girl on a safari trip. 'Oh, look! There's a big one! Look,
that one's moving! Quick! That one just opened its mouth!'

When we arrived, we asked the park ranger how much distance
we should keep between us and them.

'Oh, about ten feet,' she said languidly.

Cameron and I looked at each other. Ten feet didn't seem like
much. We'd encountered a crocodile once in Mexico and given
him a wide berth. Crocodiles were supposedly more aggressive
than alligators, but, still, an alligator could outrun a man.

We spent two days exploring the park and photographing
countless alligators. They lay sprawled in the sun, basking like
tourists at a beach resort. They lurked in the water with only their
eyes visible. They lolled half in and half out of the water, as

though unable to make up their minds. We inched as close as we dared for photographs, marvelling at their size.

On a tram ride into the River of Grass, a boy asked how many alligator attacks there had been. The guide said that since the park had opened in 1946 there hadn't been a single attack.

The boy was disappointed. 'Not even one?'

'Well, there was one incident where a kid flew off his bike into the water and landed on top of one and got bitten. But I've seen women setting their babies down on gators' backs to take pictures. You wouldn't believe the things some tourists do.'

'Are you thinking what I'm thinking?' I whispered to Cameron. 'Uh-huh.'

After the tram journey we walked back along the bank of a stream. I was looking for just the right alligator.

The ferocious deadly reptiles were as still as statues. Of course they were dangerous, but they weren't aggressive. And they surely had better things to do than eat the tourists.

'That one,' I said, pointing to an eight-footer. He was lying on the grass, facing the water. I walked right up behind the alligator and stood less than a foot from his tail. No reaction. Emboldened, I knelt beside him and gently placed my hand on the ridges of his tail, thrilling at the danger. His skin had the texture of weathered stone warmed by the sun. I turned to grin at Cameron, who was taking pictures. When I turned back to my new friend, he was slowly opening his mouth.

Hi Niki,

I think you should no longer play the naughty young girl. What I like is your appearance as a young but really adult woman. You are better in acting an adult prisoner, spy, wife, thief . . . but leave the naughty-little-schoolgirl-stuff. In movies there are better characters for you to play!

Peitschengruß,

Klingsor Whip, Stuttgart

40. HALL OF MIRRORS

It's the industry's defining image: the schoolgirl trembling before the headmaster's cane. But schoolgirls have to grow up. At least the models who play them do. There comes a time when you just can't pull off the schoolgirl act any more. Some models retire from the spotlight. Others burn out or get disillusioned. Some switch and become spankers. Others simply disappear.

In writing this memoir I've gained a new perspective. Before, the kink was just something I did, something that was part of me and needed an outlet for expression. But putting it down on paper lets me see it from the outside. The words you read here, reworked and obsessed over, paint a far more genuine picture than my fantasies and post-shoot euphoria. The words make it *real*.

When I think of the furtive cowering teenager I was, so skittish and mistrustful, I want to tell her that someday it will all make sense. Someday she'll find where she belongs. She'll never have to suffer that crushing isolation again. She'll learn to trust.

I've made so many friends in the Scene. People I trust with my life. They're the closest friends I've ever had because they know the Real Me, warts and all.

Viewers often ask what I was feeling during a particular scene. They want to know the intricacies of thought and emotion. The 'magic moment' of anticipation before the first stroke lands. The sensations afterwards.

I've answered that question many times in many ways. But the words on paper offer more insight and clarity.

Solace. That's the word that captures it best. It can't exist without the experience of pain. It's the *release* from pain. The bliss that comes from having suffered and survived. It's the culmination of a journey requiring absolute trust. The rewards are beyond measure.

Most of all I cherish the bond with the one who inflicted the pain. The one who has tamed me. In chains, I am free. There's nothing more intimate than that.

So where do I go from here? Well, my wide-eyed ingénue days are behind me, but it's refreshing to know that men like to see adult women spanked too. I must admit I've had more fun playing spies and political prisoners than schoolgirls.

The obvious next step is topping. After all, the best tops are ones who know what it's like to be a bottom. I could certainly go that route; I have my Lady Ligeia experience to draw on. But I'm not sure. There's still a part of me that will never grow up. I can always report to the headmaster again, but perhaps not in front of the camera.

One thing is certain: it's been a hell of a ride.

Sometimes the arts must transgress popular taste to allow culture to develop.

In mainstream movies, actors often perform stunts riskier than being caned. Alpine skiers sometimes die in front of the camera. I have seen it happen. It is a show for the entertainment of the masses. And the masses wouldn't watch if the skiers didn't go down that steep hill at an insane speed, accepting a calculated risk. Strangely, that is legal. If they break an arm or a leg, they are first in line in the hospital; they are heroes.

Caned women don't risk as much as that. Still, I think they too should enjoy the status of heroes.

Frants, Norway

41. MOONRISE, CHARLES BRIDGE
June 2007

The sultry night settles around me like a cloak of crushed velvet. The baroque saints along the bridge stare down at me, their faces bruised by shadows. Inscrutable.

Below, the waters of the Vltava snake their way towards the Elbe. The flickering waves sparkle like liquid stars as they whisper softly against the pillars of the bridge. Tattered clouds drift apart to unveil a dazzling full moon. All around me are the spires of old Bohemia, luminous phantoms in the eerie glow.

I couldn't stay away. I was drawn back, as though answering an ancient call.

Tomorrow, the werewolves will sink their fangs into me again. I'll suffer, cry, surrender. And float in the blissful afterglow. Pain is a lover so ardent he leaves me scarred and bleeding. He makes me suffer; he makes me feel alive.

I gaze across the bridge into the woods around Petřín Hill. Through the mist I see pinpricks of light among the trees. They might be the eyes of wolves, gleaming like unearthly candles. Watching, waiting.

If I listen with my heart I can hear them start to howl. It's a chilling sound for most, a grisly savage song. But not for me. I hear myself in that poignant howl. It awakens my wild blood like a secret sister.

It's music I can dance to. And I know every step.

Now, as then, 'tis simple truth:
Sweetest tongue has sharpest tooth.

FILMOGRAPHY

Lupus Pictures
- *Stalin 3*
- *Stalin 2*
- *Crime and Punishment*
- *Exchange Student*

pain4fem
- *The Spy*

Strictly English
- *Trial By Ordeal*
- *An American Brat in London*

RealSpankings
- *The Conspiracy*

Bars & Stripes
- *Intake*
- *Basic Instincts*
- *Silence Broken*
- *Bird of a Feather*
- *Backfire, part 1: Sting*
- *Solitary*

- *Flynn's Ordeal*
- *Backfire, part 2: Playtime*

Northern Spanking Institute
- *Cat Burglar*
- *Castigation and Caning*
- *Lessons in Latin*
- *A Ballet Beating*
- *Gymtastic!*
- *Introducing Niki Flynn*

Firm Hand
- *English School*

Websites
- Dallas Spanks Hard
- Falaka Online
- Spanked Sweeties
- Spanking Online
- Spanking Server
- Spanked Cutie

CZECH PRONUNCIATION GUIDE

A a	like u in pup
Á á	as in mama
B b	same as in English
C c	like ts in pots
Č č	like ch in chicken
D d	same as in English
Ď ď	like dy in duty
E e	as in bee
É é	like a in day
Ě ě	like ye in yes; (when it follows m: mnyeh)
F f	same as in English
G g	as in golf
H h	as in hand
Ch	like German ch in Bach
I i	as in sit; same as y
Í í	like ee in meet; same as ý
J j	like y as in yes
K k	same as in English
L l	same as in English
M m	same as in English
N n	same as in English

Ň ň	like ny in nuisance
O o	o as in dog
Ó ó	like aw in fawn
P p	same as in English
Q q	same as in English
R r	rolled
Ř ř	rolled r with ž
S s	same as in English
Š š	like sh in show
T t	same as in English
Ť ť	like ty in stupid
U u	like oo in foot
Ů ů	like oo in room
Ú ú	same as ů
V v	same as in English
W w	same as in English
X x	same as in English
Y y	like i in sit
Ý ý	same as í
Z z	same as in English
Ž ž	like s in pleasure